A Guide to the
Clinical
Interview

Daniel Levinson, M.D.

Associate Professor
Department of Family and Community Medicine
University of Arizona, College of Medicine

Illustrated by Marcia Hartsock, AMI

1987
W. B. SAUNDERS COMPANY
Harcourt Brace Jovanovich, Inc.
Philadelphia London Toronto Montreal Sydney Tokyo

W. B. SAUNDERS COMPANY
Harcourt Brace Jovanovich, Inc.

West Washington Square
Philadelphia, PA 19105

Library of Congress Cataloging-in-Publication Data

Levinson, Daniel.

A guide to the clinical interview.

1. Medical history taking.   I. Title. [DNLM:
    1. Interview, Psychological—methods. WM 141 L665g]

RC65.L48   1987   616.07′51   87–4942

ISBN 0–7216–1723–9

Editor: William Lamsback
Designer: Karen O'Keefe
Production Manager: Bill Preston
Manuscript Editor: Susan Colaiezzi-Short
Illustration Coordinator: Lisa Lambert
Indexer: Tom Stringer

A Guide to the Clinical Interview   ISBN   0–7216–1723–9

Last digit is the print number: 9   8   7   6   5   4   3   2   1

Dedicated to
My Parents

Permission to use copyrighted materials is hereby grate-
fully acknowledged to the Macmillan Publishing Company for excerpts from *Computer Applications in Clinical
Practice: An Overview*, by Daniel Levinson, M.D.

FOREWORD

The medical interview is the cornerstone of the diagnostic process. Hypothesis generation begins with initial data collection and directs the flow and content of the interview; diagnostic possibilities are considered, investigated, and maintained or refuted. Accurate and complete data collection leads to the development of a differential diagnosis and can obviate the need for expensive diagnostic procedures ordered as part of a "fact-finding mission."

The process by which the interview is conducted, the interviewer's interpersonal skills and mannerisms, is as important as the information obtained. Although a great deal of accurate data can be obtained by having the patient complete a detailed questionnaire administered by a non-physician, the invaluable nuances of the rich interaction between the physician and patient would be missed and lost. So much information can be gained by observing the patient's body language, nonverbal response to questions, and affect. An empathetic response on the part of the physician or the skillful use of a few seconds of silence can encourage the patient to reveal information not readily accessible by other means.

Good interpersonal skills also have a therapeutic value. How often we hear that the patient "feels better" just by virtue of talking to his or her doctor. Improved patient compliance in taking medication and returning for follow-up visits is also directly correlated with a physician's interpersonal skills. In this era of oversupply of physicians, there is competition for patients. It is difficult for a patient to judge a physician's clinical competence, but patients tend to judge a physician by his or her personality and the physician's ability to put them at ease and engender a feeling of trust. Interpersonal and interviewing skills are correctly perceived as vital to the patient's welfare.

I have known Dan Levinson since 1970. He is a superb physician, an accomplished interviewer, an excellent role model for students, and a kind and compassionate individual. I am so pleased that he has written this exceptional book on medical interviewing. It is a valuable resource for all of us and our students.

PAULA L. STILLMAN, M.D.
Associate Dean for Curriculum
Professor of Pediatrics
University of Massachusetts Medical Center
Worcester, Massachusetts

OVERVIEW

A skillful interview is the foundation of patient care. The interview is the primary means of establishing a *relationship* with your patient; it provides the information needed for a *diagnosis*, and often is *therapeutic.*

The interview can be studied from two perspectives—those of *content* and *technique.* Content is the information to be learned from the patient; technique refers to the personal interaction between you and your patient.

☐ Rationale and Content

To interview effectively, you must know the purpose of the interview. Clinical activities have two major goals: Problem-Solving and Health Promotion.

In a *Problem-Solving* interview, the ill patient comes to you with a problem, a set of concerns or symptoms. Your task is to translate these into a "disease definition" or diagnosis. A Problem-Centered interview addresses this clinical task.

A *Health Promotion* or Health Maintenance interview is designed to:
1. Detect early disease of which the patient is unaware.
2. Prevent disease.
3. Establish a baseline against which future observations can be evaluated.

Interviews for both types of situations obtain data related to four categories, the *Fundamental Four*:

☐ Present Illness.
☐ Past Health History.
☐ Family Health History (Hereditary/Contagious History).
☐ Personal/Social History.

The essential difference between the Problem-Centered and Health Promotion databases is the *degree* to which the data in each category are collected. The same *Fundamental Four* categories of clinical information form the framework for both types of clinical activities. In a Problem-Centered interview you are guided by the principle of *relevance*, you focus on those facts of the patient's health history that help solve the patient's problem. In a Health Promotion interview you cast a wider net to capture information that maintains health, highlights preventive measures for the patient to consider adopting, and prevents disease.

The book is divided into eight units.

Unit I: An Overview is an orientation to the health care setting, its terminology, and the basics of working with patients.

Unit II: Problem-Solving details the use of the interview as a diagnostic tool.

Unit III: Health Promotion details prevention and early detection of disease.

Unit IV: Communication Techniques describes the process of communication, both verbal (spoken) and nonverbal.

Unit V: Interview Procedures is a "how-to-do-it" guidebook to interviewing in a variety of settings.

Unit VI: Special Interviews surveys specialized and challenging situations.

Unit VII: Communication Within the Profession looks at the ways health care professionals communicate with each other.

Unit VIII: Technical Supports discusses the role of computers and other interviewing aids.

ACKNOWLEDGMENTS

This book's origins date to my meeting George Engel. I doubt I ever thought about the clinical interview before that time; certainly, I never thought of it as a serious aspect of the health care process. I have created my own variations on the basic theme I learned from Dr. Engel, but the broad outline and many of the details of my approach to interviewing are his. Dr. Engel reviewed an early draft of this book, but I doubt he will recognize parts of the finished product. Like a shipwright, a teacher does not control the destination of a ship once launched. Thus, the text is my responsibility, but I acknowledge with gratitude George Engel's many contributions to its creation. Others of the Medical-Psychiatric Liaison Group, Bill Greene especially, are represented here and remembered with pleasure.

I feel privileged to have Marcia Hartsock illustrate the book. Marcia, who has spent many years in hospital settings, has a special gift of lightening what can be somber and overly serious aspects of medicine, while still remaining respectful of both students and patients. Some of the illustrations express concepts I find are difficult for students to grasp with words alone; others reflect her perceptions of interviewing and the health care process.

Paula Stillman, of the University of Massachusetts Medical School, contributed her energies, encouragement, and many good ideas. In addition, her Patient Instructor project added an important teaching and evaluation tool.

I have been strongly influenced by Dr. Lawrence Weed, a unique and farsighted critic of the health care process. His insistence that a rational approach to clinical data is the foundation of the "art" of medicine, and a necessity if the medical profession is to realize its full potential, is reflected throughout this text.

Closer to home, H. Winter Griffith has been a major source of encouragement and good ideas. Winter's editorial judgment, wide experience, gentle suggestions, and personal friendship successfully helped me past small, and not so small, obstacles.

Angela Garcia somehow found time during her first and second years of medical school studies to critically read the entire manuscript. Her student's perspective helped me appreciate aspects of medical education I could learn no other way, and her sharp editorial eye smoothed out many rough passages.

Ruth Becker-Schaller played more of a role in the creation of this book than she realizes. Ruth is a gifted nurse practitioner and teacher, and a loving human being. Watching her with patients and with students gave me a fresh understanding of how the interview fits into the scheme of things. Also, Ruth read and criticized portions of the text.

Every aspect of our profession—whether caring for patients, doing research, or writing a book—is increasingly dependent on information resources. I am fortunate to have access to a fine medical library, the Arizona Health Science Center Library, and the help of its excellent staff. In addition to assisting in traditional library services, their MEDLINE user's course gave me the skills needed to search the medical literature from my personal computer whenever the need arose.

The staffs of the *Victim Witness* and the *Family Crisis Service* programs, two community agencies dealing with interpersonal violence, used their ingenuity and imagination (lacking money) to create an excellent approach to the interviewing process. Seeing interviewing skills used in an unfamiliar setting teaches by contrast and has been a valuable experience.

Many other persons—medical students, faculty, and friends—helped in a variety of ways. I wish I could acknowledge in detail the help given by:

Donald G. Anderson	Jerry May
Barbara Bates	Leon Michaels
Bob Berkow	Lewis Miller
Cecile Carson	Teresa Munoz
John Clochesy	David Nardone
Donna Duncan	Elaine Niggeman
Nancy Groh	Herb Pollack
Robert Heusinkveld	Elizabeth Richards
Rachel Judy	Letty Rodriguez
Hilliard Jason	Paul Rutala
Steven Kristal	Sally Watkins
Mack Lipkin, Jr.	Jane Westberg

Sumner and Leila Wolfson

Working with the staff of W. B. Saunders has been a delight. Despite the turmoil of corporate mergers and personnel turnover, they have maintained their traditionally high standards of publishing excellence. Editor William Lamsback has conscientiously guided the book at every stage. Susan Colaiezzi-Short edited the manuscript with sensitivity, excellent judgment, and good humor.

Finally, and perhaps most importantly, the patients I have cared for and the students I have helped to learn interviewing skills contributed to this book. A precept I take seriously is that of an old Hoosier philosopher who said, "It ain't the things I don't know that cause me trouble so much as the things I do know that ain't so." The interactions between physician and patient, and teacher and student, result in the constant testing of one's knowledge, and reveal that many things one knows aren't so. In this context I welcome readers' criticisms and suggestions.

DANIEL LEVINSON

CONTENTS

UNIT VII □ COMMUNICATION WITHIN THE PROFESSION

UNIT VIII □ TECHNICAL SUPPORTS

INTRODUCTION

Interview (French): "To see each other."

Webster's New Collegiate Dictionary

Interviewing, a basic clinical skill, is an interpersonal *process* intertwined with informational *content* about diagnosis, treatment, and health promotion. Process and content cannot be separated.

You rarely deal directly with *disease*, which is inaccessible, but with *illness*: the unique expression of disease in each person. Each patient's past experiences, personality, family, work, recreation, and future hopes are all part of an illness. You also deal with health promotion activities that extend life and enhance its quality. As the definition of *interview* suggests, patient and clinician interact with each other. You are not a passive recorder of information, but an essential part of the patient's experience of illness. One clinician expresses this interaction this way:

Like physicists who unintentionally influence the movement of electrons merely by turning on a light to observe them, the patient, family, and doctor cannot be detached observers. They are all involved observers affecting and being affected by the observed situation in countless ways that no laboratory test can measure. With regard to the doctor's observations, every form of diagnosis, from a kindly gaze to a complex X-ray procedure has an impact, great or small, on what it is designed to reveal. By the same token, the patient's and the family's understanding of symptoms can have a significant impact on the course of illness.

Bursztain et al, 1981

Despite the dramatic technological tools available to the medical profession, the clinical process still starts with the person-to-person interview. All that follows is determined by what you learn as you talk to the patient. A comprehensive study of medical education, *Physicians for the Twenty-First Century* (Muller, 1984), noted:

> Obtaining the history of a patient's illness is the first and most important step in evaluating the patient. Information obtained from talking with the patient usually contributes more to problem resolution than information from examination or from diagnostic tests.

Master clinicians, if asked to choose the single most valuable tool at their disposal, agree that it is the personal interview.

☐ A Systematic Approach

The approach to interviewing presented in this book is a structured, systematic one. You'll encounter the *Fundamental Four* and the *Sacred Seven*—phrases that reflect patterns that apply to all interviews. If you can remember "4" and "7," you will not get lost as you move from the beginning to the end of an interview, no matter how many side roads and detours the patient takes. A dependable framework that structures the general interview process enables you to confidently approach specific patient problems. Without a system to guide you, each patient's problem is a new experience, requiring a new approach. Daily living would be impossible without the frameworks we employ so automatically we don't even think about them.

☐ Think Organs and Systems, Not Diseases

In many medical schools, students start to interview before they have completed a course in pathology. A major concern of students just beginning to interview is their lack of knowledge of hundreds of individual diseases. In this text a disease orientation is not necessary. You will be shown an approach based on the *organs/systems* within which the symptoms are generated. There are thousands of diseases but relatively few major body organs and systems. Your premedical courses, plus first-year anatomy and physiology, are all you will need to start interviewing. (Having a major personal illness is a uniquely valuable opportunity to understand medical care, but chances are you will have to get along without this learning experience.) As you acquire more contact with patients, you will rely increasingly on pattern recognition and other nonanalytic methods, but the system-based method will never become obsolete. It will always be there to help you solve difficult problems.

A systematic approach to diagnosis requires an understanding of the *concept* of disease, however. The definition of disease used in this book will not satisfy everyone. It is offered as a practical framework within which to do the interview, conduct a focused physical examination, and obtain relevant laboratory tests—all preliminary to rational therapy.

□ Interpersonal Relationships

Interpersonal relationships are essential to the health care process. Just as a working definition of disease is needed as you begin to develop your interviewing skills, so is the awareness of the elements of interpersonal relationships. This topic is given as much attention as the "nuts and bolts" of medical diagnosis.

Wherever appropriate, the importance of patients' *lifestyle* is pointed out. Psychosocial considerations suffer relative neglect in medical education; there is so much "hard science" to be taught that the "softer" psychological and social sciences are at a disadvantage in competing for your time and attention. Decide for yourself how important such matters are. My only request is that you keep yourself open to observing psychosocial behavior as an integral part of effective health care.

This perspective, the biopsychosocial model (Engel, 1977), is a comprehensive view of the patient in health and disease. Eisenberg (1980), summarizing the transition from person to patient and back again to person, emphasizes that this movement is a function of both medical and social factors and that stress can undermine resistance to illness and disease just as support can augment it. He continues:

> ...it follows that the efficiency and effectiveness of medical evaluation will be enhanced if the physician, in assessing patient problems, regularly includes a systemic inquiry into the social determinants of the decision to seek help. Moreover, the likelihood of being able to contribute to the resolution of the human quandaries besetting the patient will be the greater the more accurately the therapeutic recommendations are directed at correcting the social determinants of the illness experience as well as at the more familiar biological components of the disease process...whether the physician wills it or not, all medical practice is a set of social and interpersonal transactions.

□ Time and Economic Realities

Fundamental changes in the economics of the health care system are influencing how medicine is practiced. Health maintenance organizations (HMOs), diagnosis related groups (DRGs), and other cost control systems, which shorten hospital stays and limit appointment time in the doctor's office, impose pressures on the time clinicians spend with their patients. Office care and home care are increasingly important parts of the overall treatment plan. These changes affect the doctor-patient relationship. The physician is changed from a patient advocate to a "gatekeeper" who determines who gets into the health care system and for how long (Korcok, 1986; Eisenberg, 1985). Rather than look back to the "good old days," clinical skills must adapt to the new economic climate. This book discusses interviewing in the office and in the home, and major attention is given the time-limited *Problem-Centered Interview*.

Finally, changes taking place in society influence health and disease and must be a part of clinical history-taking. The altered environments of the family, workplace, education, leisure, sexual behavior, and health awareness have reduced or eliminated some diseases while introducing new ones.

☐ Reasons Why

Throughout this book reasons are offered for the steps of the interview procedure suggested. This might not seem so revolutionary, but it is. Medicine is filled with traditions, and the medical interview is as traditional as any area of practice. "This is the way it is, because this is the way it has always been" exerts more influence on our clinical skills than we realize. Since the realities of a busy practice usually force the physician to select what is asked, knowing the rationale for each question is essential to obtaining a relevant history in a reasonable time.

Many of the ideas expressed in this book I've learned from others, and I have adapted them to suit my practice needs. I hope you will do the same thing. No two clinicians think in exactly the same way; there are a variety of different but successful kinds of interviews. Rigid outlines or dogmatic statements (including those in this book) should not guide your interviewing style. When you know the reasons why you do something and its relevance to the task at hand, learning is less a matter of memorization and more a natural process of growth. Throughout your medical education, ask yourself, and your teachers, "Why is this information important?" If there is no good answer, there is no reason to learn it.

This book suggests the major categories of information to ask about, and *how* and *why* to ask about them. It does not provide you with a detailed set of specific questions. No two practice situations are the same. The information you need when interviewing in a pediatric practice is different, in detail, than the information you need when in internal medicine. Similarly, other health care professional students, particularly nursing students whose education includes patient assessment skills similar to those taught to medical students, should be comfortable with this book. Part of the work of learning medicine is to adapt the interviewing framework presented in this text to the specific needs of individual specialities. The references and readings at the end of each chapter will help you.

□ Terminology

Terminology is a problem faced by everyone who learns interviewing skills. Unlike the precise, uniform labeling of the PQRST waveform of an electrocardiogram, for example, there is no standard set of terms about components of the interview. You will hear the same things referred to by a variety of terms. Terms are less important than the meaning behind them, however. The answer to the problems of terminology is understanding the *reasons why* of the interview components, whatever they are called.

□ Examples

The longer cases in the book describe patients from my clinical experience. I mistrust hypothetical cases. Each story is as accurate as condensation and the distortions of memory and personal perception allow. (Actual names and circumstances have been altered, of course.) I offer these cases to *illustrate* lessons I learned from my experience, and not as proof that they represent fundamental truths. You will have to find out for yourself. The book is a starting point from which you will discover ideas and techniques that you may find helpful.

□ Theory vs. Practice

Interviewing is a skill based on a limited set of concepts. Understanding concepts will help you get started, but don't overestimate how much help concepts are by themselves. Concepts are *word-based*; interviewing is *experience-based*. You certainly wouldn't go flying with a friend who just received an A+ on the written examination of a flying course but who had never actually flown an airplane. Word-based knowledge is, at best, a crude approximation of reality. Words acquire meaning only when associated with real-world experience. Confucius knew this long ago, when he wrote:

We hear, and we forget,
We see, and we remember,
We do, and we understand.

Use *every* opportunity to interview patients, no matter how inadequate or anxious you feel. Don't spend more time reading or watching video tapes than is necessary to learn the basics. You don't have to master interview theory before you see your first patient. Books and tapes give you answers before you know the questions. William Osler, one of the all-time great clinicians, said it all:

Medicine is learned by the bedside and not in the classroom. Let not your conceptions of the manifestations of disease come from words heard in the lecture room or read from the book. Let the word be your slave, not your master.

Becoming a skillful interviewer is mostly a matter of finding out for yourself what you need to know. "You see what you look for, you recognize what you know" is a truism that applies to all aspects of medical education and clinical practice. The more experience you have, the more skillful will you become. Learning to interview, or anything else for that matter, involves constant alternating between experience and knowledge. Too much knowledge results in intellectualization; too much uninterpreted experience results in unguided action.

Finally, don't compare your progress in learning to interview with the progress of your classmates. Learning to interview (and learning most other subjects as well) cannot be forced into a rigid time schedule or a fixed sequence of steps. Each of you will bring to the interview learning task a different background and a different learning style. Some learn rapidly, some learn slowly, but everyone can learn to be a skilled interviewer.

☐ USING A TAPE RECORDER

Observing yourself is an effective way of identifying your strengths and weaknesses as an interviewer, but you cannot monitor your interviewing performance while actually talking with someone. Direct observation by an instructor is uniquely valuable in helping you learn to interview (Engel, 1982). Some schools have facilities for videotaping you while you interview. A simple alternative is an inexpensive audio tape recorder. While an audio recording misses many of the nonverbal aspects of the interview, it is still a rich learning experience. You may be astonished to hear that you speak too fast or too quietly, use medical terms the patient could hardly be expected to understand, or ignore what the patient has told you.

The patient's permission must *always* be obtained before making any kind of recording; to fail to do so could have severe practical consequences if discovered, no matter how innocent your intent. Most patients will not object to being recorded provided they understand the reason and are assured that the tape will be erased after you have listened to it. Also, you should appreciate that any kind of recording distorts the interview to some extent, especially if you touch on sensitive topics.

A young man was admitted to the hospital because of severe colitis. He readily agreed to permit an audio tape recording, and within a few minutes seemed to forget about the recorder. Near the end of the interview, he mentioned that he was having some kind of trouble with the law. Sensing the importance of this information for the management of the colitis, the interviewer asked for more details. The patient pointed to the recorder and said, "Not while that thing is on."

□ University Settings

Most of your clinical education takes place in university health care facilities. This is another way of saying that the health care delivery system that will most strongly influence you in your formative years has its faults. University medical centers are often referral centers and are not representative of community medical practices where most people receive care. To some extent they may emphasize the technical aspects of medicine at the expense of the personal. Also, teaching centers seem to suffer from poor communications and inadequate information systems. And because of the rotations of students and residents, and faculty obligations to teaching and research, in addition to patient care, continuity of care is difficult to achieve. Considering the complexity of modern medicine and the demands of teaching and research, medical centers do a fine job. If I am at times critical of the care they provide, it is because I believe that in some ways they can and should do a better job at preparing you for the realities of practice.

□ Brevity

I value brevity (although the length of this introduction may suggest otherwise), and have tried to keep the book lean. Where possible, outlines have been used to give you an overview of a subject. With brevity comes the risk of oversimplification, but I believe that at the onset of your clinical experience you should see the broad view of a subject like interviewing, even at the expense of the errors or distortions that come with simplicity. As you acquire experience, you will modify what you learn from this book and from your instructors to acquire an interviewing style that fits your needs and perceptions. The nature of medical practice changes constantly, and I hope you will maintain in all your clinical skills the degree of flexibility needed for a fresh, innovative, and stimulating approach to patient care.

□ Books and Journals

Clinical interviewing is one subject for which you don't have to buy a lot of books. I have tried to make this text complete and practical, but you may find other books on interviewing helpful. Different authors explain the same things in different ways and appeal to different students. The following are all excellent texts:

- □ Coulehan JL, Block MR: *The Medical Interview: A Primer for Students of the Art.* Philadelphia, F. A. Davis, 1986.
- □ Enelow AJ, Swisher SN: *Interviewing and Patient Care*, Ed 3. New York, Oxford University Press, 1986.
- □ Froelich RE, Bishop FM: *Clinical Interviewing Skills*, Ed 3. St Louis, C. V. Mosby Company, 1977.
- □ Morgan WL, Engel GL: *The Clinical Approach to the Patient.* Philadelphia, W. B. Saunders Company, 1969.
- □ Reiser DE, Schroder AK: *Patient Interviewing: The Human Dimension.* Baltimore, Williams & Wilkins, 1980.

Interviewing is not a subject of extensive research, but important articles do appear regularly in leading medical journals. Some test concepts that seem to make sense, but which in fact do not prove to be so. Other articles are conceptual, personal, anecdotal, or inspirational, and usually based on the experience of one or a small group of physicians. I've tried to include references to recent, general articles, especially those with good bibliographies. Many of the references are to the literature of family medicine. This in no way suggests that this book has been written primarily for students who plan to enter family practice. Family medicine, however, has taken as its orientation health care in its broadest dimension, and its literature reflects this perspective.

The reference list is not comprehensive, and by the time this book reaches you some references will be out-dated. An up-to-date literature search requires the use of the *Index Medicus* (the MeSH heading for interviewing is "Medical History Taking"), or the impressive *Science Citation Index* for a "forward search." Skill in information management is an integral part of clinical practice (Levinson, 1978). The ability to use the medical library and, increasingly, computer-based sources of information, is an important element in success in medical school, and for the lifelong learning that will be an essential part of your professional life (Smith, 1982). After interviewing a patient, looking up the patient's condition in any standard textbook adds a valuable educational dimension. A grasp of underlying pathophysiology makes clinical phenomena more understandable. Keep in mind, however, that the "textbook picture" of any specific disease is something of a fiction—any one patient rarely manifests all of the "classic" features.

Not all the references in this text are to the prestigious journals like *The Journal of the American Medical Association* (JAMA) or *The New England*

Journal of Medicine. Popular magazines like *Discover* and *The New Yorker* often publish medical articles that, while simplified, are both accurate and enjoyable. There are also references to some "throw-away" publications such as *Medical Economics* and *Hospital Practice* that cover topics relevant to many aspects of medical practice.

Interviewing patients, while not always easy, should always be interesting and challenging. And, as the illustrations that accompany this book suggest, interviewing patients has its lighter side, at least some of the time. The effort you invest in acquiring interviewing skills should add to your sense of accomplishment during your medical school years, and will be a valuable resource throughout your career.

□ REFERENCES AND READINGS

Brody H: Ethical gatekeeping: The ongoing debate. J Fam Pract 1986; 23:539–540.

Bursztain H, Hamm RM, Feinbloom RI, et al: Medical Choices, Medical Chances. New York, Dell, 1981, pp. xx–xxi.

Eisenberg JM: The internist as gatekeeper. Preparing the general internist for a new role. Ann Intern Med 1985;102:537–543.

Eisenberg L: What makes persons "patients" and patients "well?" Am J Med 1980;69:277–285.

Engel GL: The need for a new medical model: A challenge for biomedicine. Science 1977;196:129–136.

Engel GL: What if music students were taught to play their instruments as medical students are taught to interview? The Pharos 1982; Fall:12–13.

Fein R: What is wrong with the language of medicine? N Engl J Med 1982;306:863–864

Hogness J: What about the patient? (Editorial) N Engl J Med 1985;313:689–690.

Levinson D: Information management in clinical practice. J Fam Pract 1978;7:779–805.

Levinson D: Bedside teaching. The New Physician 1970;19:729–739.

Lipkin M Jr, Quill TE, Napodano RJ: The medical interview: A core curriculum for residencies in internal medicine. Ann Intern Med 1984;100:277–284.

Muller S (chairman): Physicians for the Twenty-First Century. J Med Educ 1984;59 No 11 pt 2; entire issue.

Ransom AJ, Yager J: Future work conditions for physicians: Implications for medical education. The Pharos, 1984; Summer:12–15.

Smith MP (Project Director): The Management of Information in Academic Medicine (2 vols). Washington, Association of American Medical Colleges, 1982.

UNIT I

STUDENTS, PATIENTS, AND HEALTH CARE

CHAPTER 1

BASIC CONCEPTS

Interviewing is a practical skill based on a limited number of concepts. This chapter identifies and defines those concepts; they will be referred to many times throughout the book. Learn them and you will know the theoretic framework needed for competence as a skilled interviewer.

These concepts refer to two major areas:

1. Informational *Content*: health, illness, and disease.
2. The Interview *Process*: the technical aspects of interviewing.

☐ Health, Disease, and Illness

The interview brings you and your patient together around a concern for the patient's well-being. Six overlapping concepts apply.

Disease: A biological abnormality in structure or function.

Illness: The total experience of disease as perceived by the patient.

Symptoms: The patient's subjective, or private, awareness of disease.

Signs: Objective evidence of disease.

Sickness: Illness as a social phenomena.

Health: The optimal expression in daily living of a person's mental and physical capabilities.

☐ The Interview Process

The *interview* is a clinical tool. You use it to

1. Obtain information (*history*) from the patient that aids you in reaching a *diagnosis*.

3

2. Establish *rapport* (a working relationship) with the patient.
3. Provide some forms of *therapy*.

Interview: The process of obtaining the patient's medical history by face-to-face conversation, "to view each other."

Clinical: "At the bedside," and more generally any activity involving direct patient contact. During your clerkships you will carry out many of the duties of a *Clinician.*

History: The facts of a patient's life that are relevant to present and future diagnosis and treatment. The content of a medical history addresses four major areas (the *Fundamental Four*):
1. Present Illness.
2. Past Medical History.
3. Family Medical History.
4. Personal/Social History

Rapport: A "coming together." In general, refers to interpersonal qualities involving clear communication, acceptance, and cooperation.

Therapy: Actions that help restore a patient to optimal health.

The interview *content is* directed towards two types of clinical information:
1. Problem-Centered.
2. Health Promotion.

Problem-Centered: A limited clinical activity designed to diagnose and treat a specific problem.

Health Promotion: A clinical activity designed to:
1. Establish a *baseline* of clinical information.
2. *Detect early disease.*
3. *Prevent* disease.

A *Comprehensive* or *Complete History* combines Problem-Centered and Health Promotion information.

□ Communication Tools

Verbal (Spoken) Communication: Exchange or sharing of information by means of words.

Non-verbal Communication: Exchange or sharing of information by observable but unspoken symbols and behaviors.

Open-Ended Questions: Unstructured questions that cover broad areas of health information.

Directed Questions: Questions that seek relatively specific, detailed information.

□ Information Management

Database: Recorded data that form the informational base for care.

Mini-database: A Problem-Centered History.

Complete Database: A comprehensive or complete history.

□ Diagnostic Tools

Diagnosis: The process of identifying a patient's disease from signs, symptoms, and laboratory data.

Differential Diagnosis: Deciding which of several similar diseases is actually present.

Risk Factors: Factors in a person's Past Medical History, Family Medical History, and Personal/Social (Lifestyle) History that predispose to disease.

These definitions are not precise, and they will not satisfy everyone. The "true" meaning of terms such as *health, disease*, and *diagnosis* has been debated for centuries. Practical *working definitions* will serve our purposes. As each concept is discussed in subsequent chapters, its use in this book will be illustrated with examples. As with many other fundamental ideas that are difficult to define, you'll recognize them when you meet them.

These terms are not standard throughout the medical profession. Your instructors may use different terms to refer to the same concepts. Where possible, alternate terms are mentioned. If you understand what is being talked about, you should have no trouble translating one term into others.

□ Next Steps

This book covers basic interviewing skills. Interviewing is just one of several clinical skills you will learn before starting your clerkships. Other skills include physical examination, laboratory testing, specialty evaluations, and patient education.

Physical examination of the patient usually is guided by the history. A Problem-Centered interview is followed by a physical examination limited to the areas of relevance; a complete database, on the other hand, includes a comprehensive history and a more thorough physical examination.

CHAPTER 2

STUDENT ROLES AND CONCERNS

Can You Really Walk In And Start Interviewing A Real Patient?

Maybe you're been looking forward to clinical interviewing. When the time comes to actually meet your first patient, however, your enthusiasm may fade. Your preparation may seem inadequate. You may feel that you don't know very much about either clinical medicine or interviewing, and suspect what little you do know won't help very much.

There are perils. Suppose your patient cries—will you have somehow caused harm? Is it really fair to expect someone who is sick to participate in your education by going through a student interview? What if the patient asks you a question you cannot answer? Suppose your patient has visitors when you walk in? What do you do about patients who never stop talking, or won't talk at all, or are too confused to give you a straight answer? And what about patients who are demanding, or clinging, or seductive, or angry? Interviewing sounds like a no-win situation; you may be tempted to play it safe rather than take some chances with your ego.

Have courage. You've got more going for you than you realize. This chapter and the one following focus on your assets as a good human being as well as a student—your interpersonal skills, genuine interest in people, curiosity, and motivation to succeed. The same assets that have gotten you this far in life will help you relate to people as patients. If you can ignore the intimidating atmosphere of a large medical school and hospital, and appreciate your strengths and abilities, you'll do OK.

□ Preparation for Interviewing

You already know a good deal about the interviewing process—you made it through the Admission Committee's interviews, and you've been successfully talking to people all your life. Clinical interviewing is just specialized conversation. The difference between daily conversation and clinical interviewing is mostly in *what* you talk about; the *process* is much the same in both situations.

There really isn't a lot you need to know to interview successfully. This is one medical school course that is definitely not information-intensive. Neither is anything in this book likely to change very much next year, or 20 years from now. Instead of a lot of lecturing, reading, and memorizing, learning to interview involves mastering a few basic principles and then practicing them over and over again with patients. William Osler, one of the all-time great clinicians, said, "Medicine is learned by the bedside and not in the classroom. Let not your conceptions of the manifestations of disease come from words heard in the lecture room or read from the book. Let the word be your slave, not your master."

The simplicity of the interview format contains a hazard, however. When a task depends on a few basic principles, there isn't a lot to fall back on if something goes wrong. Reading a road map isn't very difficult, but without knowing the basics, getting lost is easy. Since the interview initiates the entire clinical process, it influences what follows: the physical examination, laboratory testing, and treatment. Mastering the basics will take both preparation and practice.

□ What Else Do You Have Going For You?

□ ROLE

Even though you are a student seeing your first patient, your name tag, white coat, stethoscope, and being a part of the system entitle you to many of the rights and privileges of a "doctor," as well as the obligations of the role. *Role* is a powerful fact of social interaction. We constantly occupy roles that define our social behaviors. Modern life would be impossible if every day we have to think through how to act in the classroom, on the tennis court, in a restaurant, making a bank deposit, getting married, or going to a funeral. In each of these and other instances, ready-made roles, learned unconsciously, define how we behave towards others, and they towards us. Since we may be strangers in many of these situations—that is, you and the other person may be meeting each other *as individuals* for the first time—each person has to identify the role being played. You may have never seen the bank teller to whom you hand over a $50 dollar deposit, but you part with your money without a second thought. The person taking the money *occupies the role* of a teller—being behind the counter, counting your money, putting it into various drawers, entering data into a computer terminal keyboard, and giving you a receipt with a smile and a parting "Have a nice day." For a delightful introduction to role theory, see Goffman (1959).

I've gone into detail about role because it defines the doctor-patient relationship that both you and your patients will understand pretty well. Most patients will unquestioningly accept you as a doctor; the problem is to be accepted as a *medical student*. Your task is to pour yourself into the role of clinician by your clothes, appearance, and sufficient knowledge of interviewing and physical examination routines so that you are comfortable with them, while at the same time modifying your role to that of medical student.

Does your status as a medical student interfere with patients' acceptance of you? Persons coming to a university medical center expect that medical students will participate in their care. Experience indicates that most patients welcome the part you play in the health care team and enjoy participating in a teaching relationship.

Will it help to introduce yourself as a "doctor" or "student doctor," or in some other way lead the patient to believe that you are not a student? This is done in some medical schools, but there are objections to the practice. The title of "doctor" carries with it obligations you cannot carry out. Suppose, for example, the patient who assumes that you are a "real" doctor asks you to prescribe a medication for sleep or some other condition, or asks for advice only the attending physician can give? It will be obvious that you seem hesitant and are unable to act on what seem to be simple requests. As a student, however, it is easy to say something like, "As a student, I cannot yet prescribe medications, but I will pass on the request to your doctor," or "That question is something that your attending doctor will have to answer." Finally, there is the possibility that allowing a patient to believe that you are a licensed physician could lead to legal difficulties. The increasingly litigious atmosphere of medical care intensifies the risk according to Oliver (1986) in an excellent article surveying the legal implications of the medical student role.

There is no reason to apologize about your student status. It is better to be viewed as an experienced medical student than an inexperienced doctor. If your preceptors advise otherwise, seek an appropriate time to discuss the question with them, or talk with your advisor or Dean of Students.

□ TIME AND INTEREST

You will often spend more time with your patients and take more genuine interest in their problems than anyone else on the health care team. Patients do form close bonds with medical students, sometimes closer than those with the attending physician.

Patients from all over the country were referred to Dr. Lester Dragstedt, one of the world's great gastrointestinal surgeons. His service consisted of a chief resident, two junior residents, an intern, two research fellows, and a medical student—me.

My first patient was a farmer from South Dakota who had been sent to Dr. Dragstedt because of intractable peptic ulcer disease. I spent many hours with him carrying out Dr. Dragstedt's pre-operative evaluation.

The afternoon before surgery the entire team visited the patient during rounds. Dr. Dragstedt assured the patient that "Everything is in order for surgery tomorrow." The only problem was that the patient's hometown doctor had somehow failed to mention that he was sending the patient to Dr. Dragstedt to have an operation—something we all assumed the patient understood.

The patient sat up in alarm, saying, "Surgery! I don't know if I want any surgery! I'll have to discuss it with my doctor."—and he pointed at me, standing at the back of the group. (The patient and I consulted. I agreed with Dr. Dragstedt about the need for the operation. All went well.)

□ Knowledge of Disease

How can you intelligently do a diagnostic interview if you don't know a great deal about disease? The answers will be explored more fully in *Unit IV: Problem Solving.* For now, a few preliminary comments. First, you already have an extensive knowledge of the body's organ systems and how they function. The diagnostic approach taught in this text is based on a *body organ/ system approach.* Even if you do not know about specific diseases, you will have no difficulty recognizing that a patient who has abdominal pain, vomiting, and diarrhea is more likely to have a disorder of the gastrointestinal tract than of the musculoskeletal system. If the patient also has chills and fever, your own health experience will suggest that the patient probably has some sort of infectious disease. Once knowing the system involved and the pathological process, what remains for a complete medical diagnosis is a bit of detective work to identify the cause or causes of the disease. You will meet the *organ/system-pathological process-cause* formula many times; it is the basis for translating symptoms and signs into a formal disease definition. Experienced clinicians seem to skip these steps and go right to the correct diagnosis, an intuitive skill that results from years of experience and learning familiar patterns. You'll develop the skill, too. At the beginning of your clinical career, however, you'll need to rely on a more deliberate analytical approach. Even the expert clinician falls back on analysis when examining a patient with an unfamiliar illness, which happens all the time, even in highly specialized practices in which you might think there is nothing new to be seen.

□ Uncertainty

Uncertainty is a stressful aspect of patient care. Unlike courses in biochemistry, genetics, microbiology, or anatomy, in which you knew what was going on with great precision, the clinical experience is filled with uncertain questions and uncertain answers. Uncertainty permeates diagnostic reasoning, treatment plans, and the entire doctor-patient relationship. When a human life is involved, is it safe to rely on such a foundation?

Your mental health and satisfaction as a clinician are linked to the kind of personal philosophy you evolve for yourself about this issue. The subject is discussed in detail in *Chapter 11: Uncertainty.* For now, the following observations may be helpful:

1. You will rarely hold the power of "life-and-death," and certainly not as a student. You are not going to kill your patients if your knowledge is less-than-perfect (perfection is an impossibility, in any event). The human body has many defenses that protect it against damage, even while sick. Over the millions of years that the human body has evolved, it has developed some cunning ways of looking out for itself. Looking back over the history of medicine, it is obvious that patients have lived *despite* the best efforts of the medical profession. Doctor Lawrence Weed, a thoughtful and intellectually honest internist, in commenting on the complexities of giving patients the correct kinds and amounts of fluids and electrolytes, observes reassuringly that, "The sickest kidney is still smarter than the smartest doctor." Everyone who has some experience in ordering intravenous fluids knows that the safest approach provides an *approximation* of total need; the patient's homeostatic mechanisms will sort out what it needs, and excrete the rest. This doesn't mean that accuracy is irrelevant, but rather than something less than perfection is satisfactory when calculating fluid balance requirements—and in most other clinical tasks as well.

2. You are not alone. Once most doctors practiced solo—alone; today doctors are a part of hospital teams and ambulatory care groups. Colleagues are constantly interacting with each other, and in so doing provide self-correcting mechanisms against error. In addition to informal chats about patients over coffee, there are more formal mechanisms: consultations, chart rounds, case conferences, and committees that look into every aspect of care. And more and more patients take part in their own care—an additional safeguard for the physician able to accept the idea that patients can monitor their own bodies.

Will you ever make an error or harm a patient? Of course you will. In a brief essay, Dubovsky and Schrier (1983) observe:

Ultimately, however, every physician must reconcile his responsibility for peoples' lives with the inevitability of making mistakes. Mistakes are distressing to the oldest as well as the youngest physician, both of whom must realize that even the most experienced and wisest of clinicians are subject to error. Indeed, clinical wisdom involves in part the acceptance of this fact. . . . This lesson is difficult to learn and difficult to teach; true self-esteem, however, is impossible when based on the necessity for omnipotence, omniscience, and infallibility. If the physician is inordinately pressured by himself or others to achieve perfection, his ability to provide and teach humaneness, as well as his personal well-being, may suffer the unhappy consequences.

As a student, you'll know how you are doing during your clerkships, not by written examinations, but by how well your work addresses your patient's clinical problems. You will learn by interacting with the other members of your clinical team. There will still be a lot of reading to do, but it will be about sick people you have interviewed and examined, not about abstract diseases.

Despite these reassurances, you will feel anxious and inadequate with some patients. You will feel overwhelmed by their problems and frustrated by the limits of present-day clinical knowledge and methods. But you learn only by getting involved and practicing. All the knowledge in the world does not substitute for actual experience, any more than reading about the theory of floating bodies will make you a swimmer. You have to jump in, even though the water is cold and uncomfortable at first. The more experience the better, even if you don't always understand everything at first. Answers make sense only when you first know what the questions are, and raw experience raises a lot of questions.

□ Patients' Participation

Is it fair to expect patients to contribute to my education? In teaching hospitals, most patients understand that they participate in the education of students—not just medical students, but also students of nursing, social work, dietetics, laboratory technique and X-ray technology, and other health care fields. At times it seems that patients are worn out by too much attention. Sometimes they are. On the day of hospital admission, a patient is interviewed and examined, in varying degrees, by the attending physician, the chief resident, and the junior resident. A student nurse has performed a nursing assessment, and a dietary student a nutritional history. Then you come along. Or maybe you are the first one to start the process. Can you possibly do anything except exhaust the patient with the kind of complete examination expected of a medical student?

There are no easy answers. Sometimes it is obvious that the patient is in no condition, physically or emotionally, to tolerate another work-up, however well-intentioned and considerate you may be. If this is your assessment, discuss the situation with the team resident. Often your assignment can be postponed, to everyone's relief. But other times your interview, even if causing some stress, will help, not hurt. And usually, your assigned patients will welcome you, especially

□ Patients who are "uninteresting" medically, and relatively neglected.
□ Patients who are bored and have nothing to do while recovering.
□ Persons who take a genuine interest in helping you in your medical education.
□ People who like to talk about themselves.
□ People who tell you things about themselves no one else seemed

interested in: their family, work, hobbies, and life philosophy. Your attention makes them feel important, something they may lack in their daily lives. Often the final thing a patient will say as you leave is "Thank you"—not just in a polite, social way, but with warmth and appreciation.

Patients contribute to our education all of our professional lives. No two patients with the same diagnosis are ever exactly the same. There is no such thing as an "uninteresting patient." Your patients will come from life settings and circumstances you'd never have a chance to learn about any other way than in medical practice. And almost always both you and your patients will benefit from the relationship.

□ Adding New Knowledge

Not only are you well-prepared to begin seeing patients, but you are in an excellent position to make original, useful contributions to medical science. You may observe clinical conditions that no one has seen before, or at least recognized as something novel and worth investigating. The impressive knowledge base of modern medicine is just a small fraction of what is yet to be discovered. Experienced clinicians know that present knowledge about health and diseases is limited. No satisfactory diagnosis is established for some patients despite thorough work-ups. And many patients with perplexing illnesses get well just as mysteriously as they got sick. Thirty years from now you will look back with amusement at some current medical concepts, just as we smile at the state of medical knowledge of the 1950's. A vast amount remains to be learned about familiar diseases, and altogether new disease will be identified. Think of the newly identified diseases of the past few years: AIDS, toxic shock syndrome, Legionnaires' disease, Reye's syndrome.

While I don't suggest that you start your clinical experience anticipating a Nobel Prize by the time you graduate, I do hope you will develop a healthy skepticism about what you read and hear. Keep in the back of your mind experiences that just don't make sense to you. Maybe they don't make sense because current explanations are wrong or incomplete. Maybe we are making things harder for ourselves than they really are. Truly significant understanding, like the double helix of DNA, has an elegant simplicity when all the false leads and misconceptions drop away. As students you are better equipped for original clinical observation than many experienced clinicians who accept through familiarity the current framework of medical knowledge. A rustic Hoosier philosopher once commented on the state of his scientific knowledge: "It ain't the things I don't know that cause me trouble so much as the things I do know that ain't so."

□ Conclusion

This chapter addresses the almost universal medical student feeling of inadequacy. Despite your academic and personal achievements, if you are like most students, you will feel lost, insecure, perhaps a bit frightened, as you begin your patient contacts. Yet the only way to learn is to practice bravely—to take chances on making mistakes. The risks are not great, but they will seem great.

Despite all of these reassurances, you will still find yourself feeing inadequate, especially as you look around and see other students, residents, and attending physicians who go about their duties with obvious self-confidence and poise. All is not as it seems, however.

Not long ago, during a recession, the physicians in one city were hard hit. The major factory had shut down, and patients were staying away if at all possible.

One physician was having a particularly hard time. He had just opened up his office and had not yet built up a practice large enough to earn even his expenses. He needed another source of income, but mindful of his status, felt he could not take just any job. Then he heard about a part-time opportunity at the zoo.

The zookeeper explained that a lion had died and the zoo could not afford to replace it. But they had saved the skin, and if the doctor would be willing to get into the skin and parade inside the cage when he had some free time, no one would know, and he could earn a few needed dollars.

The next afternoon the doctor donned the suit and climbed into the lion cage. It was a sunny day, the children seemed to believe he was a real lion, and all in all the job was working out. Suddenly, however, out of the corner of his eye, the doctor saw that there was another lion in the same cage, and it was headed in his direction. In a panic, he started to call for the zookeeper when the other lion arrived at his side, and said, "Shut up, you fool. I'm a doctor, too."

□ REFERENCES AND READINGS

Dubovsky SL, Schrier RW: The mystique of medical training. JAMA 1983; 250:3057–3058.

Feinstein AR: What kind of basic science for clinical medicine? N Engl J Med 1970; 283:847–852. (Responding letters: N Engl J Med 1971; 283:339–341.)

Goffman E: The Presentation of Self in Everyday Life. New York, Doubleday, 1959.

Oliver R: Legal liability of students and residents in the health care setting. J Med Educ 1986; 61:560–568.

SEEKING AND ACCEPTING MEDICAL CARE

Why do people seek care? The obvious answer, "To get well and stay well," suggests that people have a clear understanding of sickness and health and know when they need medical help. This is true only in clear-cut situations such as injuries or severe pain. For lesser degrees of disability or discomfort, and even more for prevention and health maintenance, wide differences among people influence their entry into the health care system. The same diversity exists when a diagnosis has been made and treatment begins. Fortunately, most patients' behavior is straightforward: their problem is clear, their course uncomplicated, and you enjoy the satisfaction of seeing that what you learn in medical school really works and really helps people. Other patients, however, will puzzle you: nothing seems to be the way you were taught. A practice of all "easy" patients lacks challenge; a practice of all "difficult" patients is frustrating. Fortunately, most practices have some of each.

☐ ILLNESS BEHAVIOR

Illness—the experience of disease—creates a series of possible responses. Some make things worse. What people do when sick will at times bewilder you. "Hidden agendas" (Barsky, 1981) will throw you off balance. Sometimes an antagonistic doctor-patient relationship, which neither you nor the patient want, develops and worsens things.

When people are ill, behaviors other than conventional medical care are possible.

Self-treatment. The most common response by far is self care. We have symptoms all the time that we know will go away by themselves or with (and sometimes despite) simple remedies offered by the over-the-counter drug industry. Patient education programs and materials extend the scope of responsible self-care.

Denial. A symptom represents a threat with which the patient cannot cope. Denial removes the symptom from awareness, and relieves the patient of anxiety and fears.

Mr. Epson, a 42-year-old accountant, was an intense, driving man. It was no surprise when his wife called about her husband, who was having severe chest pain, pallor, and marked sweating—almost certainly a heart attack. An ambulance was ordered, and I went to the emergency room to meet the patient and expedite care. The ambulance backed into the unloading area, and I opened the door. No patient! Then I heard a voice, "I'm up here, Doc." By the time the ambulance had arrived the pain was less severe, and the patient insisted on riding up front with the driver. Throughout his hospitalization, and afterwards, Mr. Epson, who was not a disagreeable person, did little to help the doctors and nurses—saying, in effect, "I'm really not sick."

Cancer and heart disease are two common threats that lead to denial. A woman who finds a breast lump, for example, may make an appointment for a "check up" and not mention the breast mass at all, on the theory that if cancer is present you'll find it. If you say nothing, she concludes she doesn't have cancer.

Sometimes patients are correct in their suspicions of serious disease, but incorrect about the meaning of the disease. Often early diagnosis and treatment lead to cure. The tragedy of denial is the time lost, and with it the opportunity for prevention or cure.

☐ SEEKING HELP

Deciding to get medical help for an illness is no casual matter. Making an appointment often is the final step in a pathway of demographic, psychological, social, cultural, and practical factors. Some people want care for mild symptoms, whereas others tolerate a good deal of discomfort; some ethnic groups have great faith in doctors whereas others turn to spiritual or folk resources; some cultures encourage entry into the sick role, whereas others discourage it. In addition, everyone has some sort of "health belief system" (Becker et al, 1977) whose components include judgments (right or wrong) about personal vulnerability, the seriousness of the possible underlying condition, and how likely is medical care to make any difference.

A woman in her 50s had for some years endured a painful knee condition,

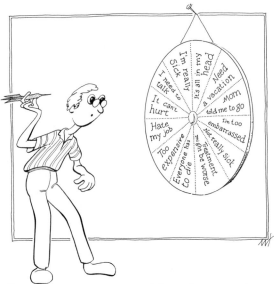

Deciding to get medical help for a problem
is often no casual matter.

affecting both knees and causing a marked walking impairment. Various treatments produced only temporary relief, and gradually she came to accept the condition.

One day she heard in glowing terms about joint replacement surgery from a physician. She went to a medical center where this type of therapy was well-advanced. She met all the criteria for joint replacement, and underwent treatment of both knees. Two months later she was pain-free, and within a year the limp had disappeared.

Current events may result in a patient seeking your help.

A 42-year-old man, a Democrat and admirer of President John Kennedy, was deeply affected by the assassination. He was interested in the neck wound and tried to visualize the bullet's course from what he had read. A day or two later he developed definite tightness in the neck.

Keeping an eye on television and the newspapers may help you anticipate the kinds of problems a few patients will suddenly develop. AIDS, for example, because of its relationship to covert sexual behavior, has already resulted in reports in the literature describing "AIDS Anxiety" (Frolkis, 1986). Also, terrorists' threat to poison a city's water supply, or the poisoning of commercial products, can trigger symptoms in suggestible persons prone to hysterical behavior.

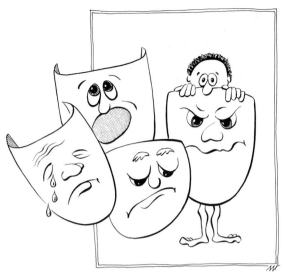

People come to the doctor wearing masks
that conceal their true feelings.

The need for more information about what is *causing* their problem, and whether the symptom represents something serious, is a common reason that people go to a doctor. A patient may not want a thorough diagnostic work-up or treatment. If reassured that the condition is not serious, or is something that is "going around" and will soon cure itself, many people are content to stop there and give the problem more time. They are satisfied with your just giving the condition a name or receiving a simple biological explanation. They then feel in control of something they understand, rather than anxious about something they don't. Misreading a request for information as a request for treatment converts a minor condition into one with potential for complications. Starting an extensive evaluation entangles the patient in expense and inconvenience, and prescribing medications may cause side effects. If, at the end of an evaluation, nothing shows up, or the medication hasn't worked, you are left with someone who now worries because the cause of the symptom cannot be found. Indeed, the anxiety created causes the patient to pay more attention to the symptom, which may worsen for this reason alone. Knowing when to reassure and when to pursue a full evaluation depends on experience, judgment, and your willingness to tolerate a degree of uncertainty. This is why you have preceptors to guide you.

Finally, there is the group of patients who want help but don't quite come out and say so. They may worry that they will be ridiculed if they state their need openly. So they complain of something like a pain, which they feel doctors accept as a legitimate reason for a visit, when in fact they are really worried about some other matter involving guilt, shame, a personal weakness, or failure. Most people are strongly motivated to maintain self-esteem at any cost (Rochlin, 1973) and cannot admit personal qualities that go against the virtues of strength, self-reliance, and success. So people come to their doctors wearing masks that conceal true feelings and needs. When rapport exists, they quit pretending. Such trust takes time, and it develops only after testing you to find out how accepting you are of a person's weaknesses.

☐ HIDDEN AGENDAS

Patients seek medical care for many reasons other than those already listed. If you misread the reason, your initial response may not address the true, rather than the surface, situation. Motivations for coming for care are varied:

Family pressures. "If you don't see a doctor *tomorrow* about your weight and smoking, I'm taking the children and leaving you. I don't want to be a young widow!"

Disability qualification. Payments by insurance companies and many social agencies depend on medical verification of a person's continuing disability.

Administrative purposes such as being excused from work or school, sometimes after-the-fact.

Permission or approval. Sometimes the patient needs a doctor's OK or approval, but doesn't know it. Sometimes writing out a prescription for a harassed housewife to hire a baby sitter or have one night out a week for dinner or a movie is wonderful therapy. (Giving advice is another matter. This will be discussed in a later section.)

Loneliness. The physician, or the physician's staff, may be the patient's only source of human contact, kindness, or advice or the only outlet for bottled-up feelings. A "visit to the doctor" is a social occasion that provides brief but valued relief from an otherwise isolated life. McPhee (1984), in a lengthy article in *The New Yorker* detailing the problems seen in a Maine family practice, describes the following:

Fifty-nine-year-old female, in slacks and running shoes, says she has come in to discuss her arthritis. Her gnarled fingers sparkle with gemstones. After a time, the doctor says "So for now you want to stick with aspirin?" He knows, though, that she is not here to talk about aspirin, or even her chronic headaches, for which she takes Elavil. She is here just to talk, as she has been in the past and will be in the future, and he is more than prepared to listen. Two relatives of her husband live at home; each is retarded and needs special care. As time has passed, the situation has grown less tolerable to her. There is nothing the doctor can prescribe except his time, his interest, and his watchful sympathy—all of which she receives.

Confession. Barsky cites a man who made repeated visits for various urogenital complaints. Examinations disclosed no evidence of disease, but the patient continued to have complaints. The problem, it turned out, was guilt about having visited a prostitute: he needed to confess to someone.

Having looked at reasons people seek help, you might suppose that once you've made your way through the maze of denial and hidden agendas and arrive at a valid diagnosis, that treatment will be a breeze. Not always so. Two areas remain to be negotiated: (1) sick role behavior, and (2) adherence to the treatment plan.

□ SICK ROLE BEHAVIOR

Being sick in most cultures confers benefits, at least temporarily, on the individual. The sick role, as defined by Parsons (1951), has four characteristics. The patient:

1. Is excused from normal responsibilities.
2. Did not want to be sick and cannot get well by personal effort alone.
3. Has the obligation to leave the sick role as soon as possible.
4. Must obtain and cooperate with a socially accepted health care provider in getting well.

Most people enter and leave the sick role appropriately. For some, however, being sick has more psychosocial benefits than being healthy. Being sick brings out in others a caring attitude that is not given when well. Basically dependent, immature persons find sickness a psychologically successful coping mechanism, whatever the cost in self-esteem and normal gratifications. And some persons, whose lives have been filled with disappointments and over-whelming obstacles, lose the courage to go on. A trivial event, such as a minor accident at work, triggers a massive withdrawal into sickness. Such persons unconsciously frustrate every effort to restore them to health. These patients are not aware of the factors that create and maintain their sick role behavior. (True malingering, in which someone consciously and deliberately assumes the sick role, is quite rare, however.) Such patients genuinely act out their parts, and expect you to do your part, too. To openly question whether they are *really* sick meets with outright hostility. Whatever rapport exists is destroyed, and with it the chance to help the patient, over the long run, to reach the best possible adjustment.

Whatever the facts about each patient's gains and losses in being sick, all must enter into a relationship with a socially recognized healer who validates their sick role status. This is where you come in. You will find yourself, as a medical student, one of the cast of characters in the patient's enactment of the sick role. In this context, the interview consists of more than a quick, "Where does it hurt?" type questioning. Instead, you find yourself, to a greater or lesser degree, involved in patients' life setting. Personal relationships, work, recreation, and personal habits all enter into the total "getting sick/getting well" equation.

Active cooperation in carrying out the treatment plan is the other component of illness behaviour that seems obvious, but is not. Patients don't always do what is in their own best interests, despite a genuine wish to abandon the sick role as soon as possible. Non-adherence, or non-compliance (an unfortunate but entrenched term that implies a *passive* patient role in an authoritarian doctor-patient relationship), is mostly a matter of not taking medications, but also includes neglecting recommended diets and ignoring a wide variety of preventive behaviors. The patient's health beliefs, mentioned previously, play an important role, as do practical matters such as having the money to fill an expensive prescription. A final determinant is how well the doctor-patient relationship has developed and been nutured, how well you have "read" the patient. More about this issue will be discussed in Chapter 4, but it has been well summarized by Zola (1981):

> ... part of what patients are responding to when they do not cooperate is not the medical treatment but how they are treated, not how they regard the required regime but how they themselves are regarded. Unless we fully recognize this phenomena, we will live out the warning of Walt Kelly's immortal Pogo, "We have seen the enemy, and they is us!"

☐ CONCLUSION

People come (or don't come) to doctors for a wide variety of reasons, which are difficult to guess. Missing the hidden agenda, like making a wrong turn in unfamiliar country, leads to wasted time and money and generates strong emotions. Other chapters of this book will help you pick up the clues patients almost always give about their true, but not openly expressed, needs. To successfully understand your patients involves going beyond a narrowly defined disease orientation. Your success as a clinician will at times require that you

> ... develop an understanding of the meaning of specific symptoms to the patient and the influence of the social setting on shaping the experience of illness. Along with choosing drugs, procedures, and services to meet the identified biomedical needs, the physician should negotiate an approach to these interventions that is appropriate to the expectation priorities, and resources of the patient and his or her family. The goal is an integrated "biopsychosocial" approach to patient problems that responds to the subjective reality of illness as well as the objective reality of disease (McKay et al, 1984; Engel, 1980).

□ REFERENCES AND READINGS

Barsky AJ: Hidden reasons some patients visit doctors. Ann Intern Med 1981;94(Part 1):492–498.

Becker MH, Haefner DP, Kasl SV, et al: Selected psychosocial models and correlates of individual health-related behaviors. Med Care 1977;15:27–46.

Engel GL: The clinical application of the biopsychosocial model. Am J Psych 1980;137:535–544.

Ford CV: The Somatizing Disorders. Illness As A Way of Life. New York, Elsevier Biomedical, 1983.

Frolkis JP: "AIDS" anxiety. Postgraduate Med 1986;79:265–576.

Klass P: How sick is it to want to be sick? Discover 1986; Jan:20–22.

McKay DA, Gill DG, Cowill JM: Sociocultural influences on medicine and health. *In* Rakel RE (ed): *Textbook of Family Practice*, ed 4. Philadelphia, W B Saunders Co., 1984, pp. 215–225.

McPhee J: A reporter at large: Heirs of general practice. The New Yorker July 23, 1984:40–85.

Rochlin G: Man's Aggression: The Defense of the Self. New York, Dell Publishing, 1973.

Zola IK: The case of non-compliance. *In* Eisenberg L, Kleinman A (eds): The Relevence of Social Science for Medicine. Boston, D. Reidel Publishing Company, 1981, pp. 241–252.

CHAPTER 4

RAPPORT AND THE CLINICAL INTERVIEW

Daniel Levinson, M.D.
Robert E. Rakel, M.D. *

The clinical process, reduced to its essentials, consists of diagnosis and then treatment. With some clinical conditions a computer could interact with the patient, make a correct diagnosis, and come up with the right treatment. But for most people and most illnesses, a human element—the clinician—must enter the picture for optimal, satisfying health care. No computer can begin to perform the spectrum of tasks the clinician does routinely. And beyond the clinician's superior technical abilities, there enters the powerful, uniquely human element of *rapport* (literally, to bring together). The human relationship between doctor and patient is the arena within which personal interactions take place—relationships that make or break the effectiveness of health care.

☐ The Value of Rapport

Rapport adds to the effectiveness of each aspect of the clinical process. During the interview, it gives your patients the courage to disclose intimate,

---

*Professor and Chairman, Department of Family Medicine, and Associate Dean for Academic and Clinical Affairs, Baylor College of Medicine, Houston, Texas.

22

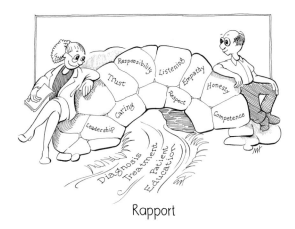

Rapport

sensitive facts about themselves that they will share with no one else. During the physical examination, rapport helps the patient through times of embarrassment or discomfort. Rapport is an essential element of therapy, promoting a cooperative attitude, adherence to treatment, and continuity of care. Rapport with the patient's family enlists their help in compiling the medical history and their positive contributions to care. Finally, rapport with the people you work with as a team encourages efficiency, optimal functioning, and personal satisfaction.

□ Communication and Rapport

Just exactly what this human quality of rapport is cannot be fully defined in words—it has to be experienced. But whatever rapport is, communication is the key to putting it into practice. Adapting the communication skills you already have to the clinical setting is what much of this book is about.

Communication is an exchange of information over some type of channel. In the clinical setting, the face-to-face conversation is the primary channel. (The telephone is an important secondary communication channel in clinical practice, and will be discussed in a later chapter.) If you live in an area where a large segment of the population speaks a language other than English, you will find acquiring a workable knowledge of that language a great investment in establishing rapport, as well as in simply getting necessary information.

□ Empowerment

For clinical communication to occur, both persons in the communication channel must have information to contribute. One-way communication has a place—in patient education materials, for example—but is less powerful than two-way interaction. In terms of establishing rapport, meaningful two-way communication is essential.

Empowerment refers to those actions you take that enable the patient to communicate with you. Most people come to a physician in a needy, dependent state. They are ill, and self-care attempts have failed to relieve the situation. Further, many patients have little detailed knowledge of medicine. In other words, they are in your power.

Given patients' dependent situation, you must encourage them to communicate fully. In a sense, they will "speak only when spoken to," unless you take the initiative. Passive patients rarely benefit fully from health care; some create real problems because you do not really understand their needs, and they just don't have the courage to speak up. If, however, you make a deliberate effort to include patients as active participants in their health care, many will respond with gratifying enthusiasm. Some techniques of empowerment, leadership and active listening, for example, are discussed in other sections of this chapter.

□ Listening Well

A good physician must be a good listener. Of all the communication skills essential to good rapport, *listening well* is among the most important. Concentrating on what your patient wants to tell you opens up a communication channel. Listening is more than silence (although silence is sometimes a powerful way of listening), it is the hard work of searching for meaning on several levels, while also providing encouragement and guidance.

Listening as a principle of good interviewing may strike you as paradoxical. Taking an active lead, rather than listening, seems intuitively what you should be doing. And you do have a lot to say; you just can't sit there and listen. While there are emergencies in which realistically you don't have much time to listen, in most practice situations, and certainly in your clerkships, time is available if you make it a priority.

Dr. Brown, a fine, respected physician with a thriving practice, had the admirable quality of always seeming to have time to listen to his patients. He used a habit developed while interning in an extremely busy county hospital. Each morning he divided the number of minutes available for his rounds by the number of patients he needed to see. Usually, he had six or seven minutes for each patient. At each patient's bedside, he sat down, relaxed, and focused all of his attention on that patient for the time available. Somehow, six or seven minutes of undivided attention was more satisfactory for both the patient and the doctor than the usual rounds where the physician, standing at the bedside, glances through the chart, asks a few questions, maybe does a brief examination, and edges towards the door.

The kind of listening we are talking about is more an *attitude* than a word count—an attitude that keeps you open to what the patient tells you, even if it doesn't fit your preconceptions. It is a fundamental shift from an authoritarian, "I'll ask the questions, you just answer 'yes' or 'no'" to an attitude of "Tell me more about. . . ." More will be said about "open-ended" attitudes in interviewing techniques in following chapters.

Studies of doctor-patient interactions indicate clinicians talk much more than do their patients (although they believe it is the other way around). Korsch and Negrete (1972) studied 800 interactions between physicians and parents in a pediatric clinic. Their findings indicated that not listening had a negative affect on several aspects of care. For example, 26 percent of mothers said they had not mentioned their greatest concern about their child because they had not been given the opportunity or encouragement by the doctor to do so. Nearly half the mothers left the clinic without learning from the doctor what had caused the child's illness; many incorrectly blamed themselves. Cooperation in adhering to the treatment plan was linked to the mother's satisfaction with the visit. The investigators concluded, "However well informed a physician may be, and however conscientious about applying his knowledge, if he cannot get his message across to the patient, his competence is not going to be helpful."

Similar findings were reported by Beckman and Frankel (1984) in a primary care internal medicine clinic. They studied how residents responded to patients' initial statement of their problems, the chief complaint. Of 74 office visits, in only 23 percent were patients allowed to finish their opening statement. Most of the patients, 69 percent, were interrupted before finishing a full statement of the reason for their visit.

Other problems with listening have been observed: distorting the patient's history to fit some preconceived typical pattern, conducting interviews so as to minimize the patient's participation in decisions such as having major surgery, and missing altogether the true reason (the hidden agenda) for a patient's visit (Waitzkin, 1984; Barksy, 1981).

You don't have to study medical settings to appreciate the value of listening. Successful salespeople at the corporate level do not talk executives into buying; they listen attentively to discover a need their product can fill.

□ Empathy

Empathy is your capacity to understand and participate in the feelings of the patient, while at the same time retaining the objectivity needed to be of optimal help. Empathy is based on having insight into what your patient is experiencing. Having been seriously ill yourself, or sharing in the care of a family member or close friend who is ill, provides a sense of empathy obtainable in no other way. Your capacity to appreciate your patient's situation diminishes the isolation created by illness, and the fear that "no one knows what is really

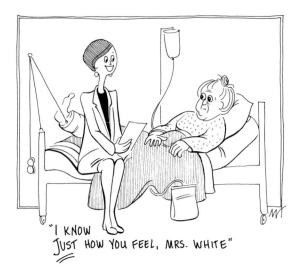

"I KNOW JUST HOW YOU FEEL, MRS. WHITE"

Be cautious about expressing empathy.

happening to me." Be cautious about expressing empathy, however; there are some illness experiences you cannot understand.

Being in touch with the patient without becoming entangled in a sympathetic emotional reaction is difficult. The last thing a distressed patient needs is a distressed caretaker. But some situations have a strong influence on our feelings despite our resolve to remain objective, as reflected in the following episode:

A second-year medical student was interviewing a faculty member simulating a depressed patient. As the interview proceeded, the student seemed increasingly caught up in the situation, forgetting that the interview was a role playing exercise and that her classmates were observing. As the simulated patient continued his history, the question of suicide was raised. Suddenly the student broke into tears and said she couldn't go on. She had a brother with a long history of depression, including a suicide attempt, and the family's efforts to help him had not been particularly effective. Now the family was telling her, "You're in medical school. You should know what to do."

This reaction occurred in a classroom setting. Think of the stress that occurs when caring for real patients with whom you have things in common.

Reiser and Rosen (1984) illustrate the empathy/sympathy process of "too close" and "too distant" as a dynamic, changing one:

Imagine that a doctor is interviewing a young woman in her twenties hospitalized for a flare-up of her diabetes that worsened after her mother died a month before. The patient's lips begin to quiver, and tears well up in her eyes. The doctor, in turn, feels himself growing teary eyed and momentarily fears that he too will burst into tears. He draws back and regards his patient for a moment from a safer distance. Quickly regaining his composure, he almost instantaneously draws closer again and says softly, "You miss her terribly, don't you?" The patient now sobs openly.

□ Leadership

An issue closely related to caring is *leadership*—the way you direct your patient's care. Traditionally, most clinicians have been authoritarian in the doctor-patient relationship: doing most of the talking, asking "yes-or-no" questions, and telling the patient what to do and how to do it. This model is still suitable in many clinical situations; certainly, an emergency room with a seriously injured patient is no place for open-ended reflection and negotiation. But in most clinical settings there are less authoritarian options. The degree to which patients successfully accept and cooperate with you in treatment ("compliance") often reflects the degree to which they participate in the treatment decisions. The trend of American society is away from a rigid social structure, as reflected in the women's movement and insistence on equal rights for all groups. The medical profession is moving in this direction. Some clinicians, rather than directly telling the patient what to do, negotiate a "therapeutic contract," especially for long-term conditions such as weight control and altering maladaptive behaviors that require the patient to take considerable responsibility if improvement is to occur. Educating patients about their bodies and their illnesses is a significant trend to comprehensive health care.

To sum up questions of acceptance and leadership, the catalyst concept may be useful. A catalyst is an agent of change, facilitating chemical reactions that are inherent in the nature of the reacting substances without being altered itself. In some situations, particularly psychotherapy, the clinician's role may be that of a catalyst—helping people achieve for themselves the best health of which they are capable. In other situations, the physician participates directly in bringing about change. A surgeon, for example, actively intervenes to stop a hemorrhaging wound or remove an inflamed appendix. In most instances, however, the physician has considerable power, but cannot be effective unless the patient is an active participant. Exercising power wisely means giving the patient substantial responsibility for seeing therapy through to a successful conclusion.

□ Touch

Touching the patient, whether a simple handshake, a part of the physical examination or treatment, or expressing deeply felt emotion, has always been an integral part of medical care. Touch is a powerful form of communication. The "laying on of hands" may promote healing, especially if it is imbued by the patient with symbolic value. Franz Mesmer (1734–1815) sometimes achieved remarkable results by what he liked patients to believe was the magnetic power of his hands—he "mesmerized" them. Today, touch as a clinical technique receives little or no attention in medical education, although twelve medical schools world-wide offer courses in physical contact (Older, 1984).

Exercise good judgment, however. The extent to which you include touch as a part of your relationship with patients is highly individual; there are no rules other than your good sense. Be alert to the patient's attitudes and social norms. Appropriately and spontaneously, a squeeze of the arm, holding a hand, even a hug, can be a powerful component of rapport, especially when a good relationship has existed for some time. But there are hazards, however pure your intentions. One attorney warns

I have unsuccessfully defended physicians on several occasions when a patient misunderstood their intentions. Apparently the patient didn't think that the hug, kiss, or knee pat was fatherly at all. When a second or third hug or kiss occurred, a lawsuit followed.

(Griffith, 1985)

□ Personal Characteristics

□ AGE

Age is one factor in establishing rapport. All other things being equal (which they never really are), more years suggest more experience, ability, maturity, even wisdom. Occasionally a youthful appearance interferes with rapport.

Dr. Morton was a capable, experienced cardiologist who appeared even younger than his actual age of 36. Among his patients was a man in his 60's—a garrulous, fiercely independent farmer who had his first hospitalization ever for a myocardial infarction. He was initially cared for by his family physician, but when a potentially dangerous arrhythmia developed a week after the infarction, he was transferred to Dr. Morton at the University Hospital.

The patient had never accepted the fact of his infarction, and as soon as the pain stopped he began to deny that there was anything wrong with his heart. He imagined that the doctors were just after his money. When Dr. Morton appeared, the patient's suspicions deepened. Dr. Morton looked too young to be a doctor, much less a specialist.

The day following the patient's admission to Dr. Morton's cardiology service, the housekeeper came in the room to clean. The patient asked her, "Have you ever heard of a Dr. Morton?" The housekeeper said she had not.

The patient put on his clothes and left the hospital.

Three days later, while pitching hay, he suffered a second infarction, which he barely survived. He was very happy to see Dr. Morton on this admission.

There are a few things you can do if you think you look "too young" even to be a medical student. If you sense that your patient has trouble accepting you, discuss the situation. Find a way to tactfully ask if your youth is a problem for the patient, and listen carefully for the true situation. Briefly explain your educational background. Maybe the concern is that you are to be the *only* doctor, when the patient expected to be under Dr. Smith's care. The patient may not come right out and say so—most people are too kind for that—but whatever the problem, if you listen, you will find out and know how to deal with it. Your openness itself will communicate your maturity.

Conservative dress also helps your professional image. Men can grow a beard (and perhaps stroke it occasionally when deep in thought). A too-youthful-appearing woman might tie her hair into a bun. Usually, however, age will not be a significant problem in your student role.

□ PERSONAL APPEARANCE

Appearance communicates a great deal about you, and influences whether you and your patient get off to a good start. A professional appearance makes a good first impression, and first impressions are important. Just what is "professional appearance" these days is hard to say. Some medical schools have a dress code, others don't. Whether to wear a shirt and necktie, or a dress, often is left to your own judgment. You are not likely to go wrong by erring on the side of formality. Many patients have conventional ideas about what a doctor should look like. They may have trouble accepting you in blue jeans and jogging shoes (Dunn et al, 1985). No one will mind if you are dressed up a bit, and most will take it as a sign of respect. In practice, once you and your patients have a secure relationship, dress is less important.

One element of appearance about which there is no disagreement is cleanliness and neatness. Sometimes, under the pressures of long hours of study and work, standards slip. Unhappily, "Not even your best friend will tell you," to quote a popular advertisement a few years ago for a deodorant soap. Many medical schools have locker rooms where you can shower and keep a supply of deodorants, talcum powder, and a toothbrush. If your school doesn't, look around; you can almost always find a way to freshen up when you need to. And the ad is right; no one, not even your best friend, is likely to have the courage to tell you when you do have a problem.

□ PLEASANT MANNER

A smile and a pleasant manner are valuable assets anywhere, and certainly in a medical setting. A smile reflects inner pleasure. . . and creates it. An Olympic Ski Team coach taught what he felt to be the key to championship performance: "Breathe and smile at the same time." It works, at least while skiing. You cannot be tense while breathing and smiling as you head down a steep slope. As for aiding rapport, think over your own experiences with others to get an idea of how a pleasant manner may help a relationship. For the stresses—minor and major—that are a part of daily practice, the motto "be of good cheer" helps things go much easier.

A pleasant personality in the absence of competence, however, is hollow, even dangerous. But competence alone is not adequate. Patients and staff may tolerate a tactless, insensitive physician of outstanding ability, but such relationships are characterized by friction, anxiety, anger and, sooner or later, disloyalty.

□ HONESTY

Honesty is essential to rapport. Truth-telling sometimes raises difficult questions in practice, however. Ethical problems will come up many times during your clinical clerkships. For now, just one brief comment.

A problem you may face—most students do—relates to your knowledge and responsibilities. An unenlightened educational experience in the past, or perhaps an overly demanding home, may have so conditioned you to an expectation of perfection of knowledge and performance as to invite dishonesty. A slight pause, "Well, . . ." or qualifiers like, "I think that . . . " are clues to the true state of things. Whether or not others consciously recognize your hedging, they weaken confidence and trust. Perfection is unattainable, and not worth the price if it were. "I don't know the answer to that" or, "No, I have not yet completed the assignment" has a quality of simplicity that commands respect and strengthens rapport (Herwig, 1986).

□ COMPETENCE

"How competent are you"? is in the minds of some patients. You can't just come out and *tell* them that your are competent. If you had your own office and a wall full of diplomas and certificates, it would help; but you have neither.

Actually, many patients don't give the question any thought. A white coat or a stethoscope is enough validation. The real challenge is mastering the tasks appropriate to your student role.

A well-organized idea of what you are doing communicates competence. Having to step out to get forgotten writing materials or examination instruments, or not knowing the interview procedure and fumbling through your notes, undermines your patient's confidence. This doesn't mean that you cannot afford to ever make a slip. It's a matter of degree. As you become more comfortable in the clinical setting, and as your skills mature, so will your confidence, which will be communicated in everything you do.

□ Professional Philosophy

□ POSITIVE REGARD AND RESPECT

Whatever your view of the helping relationship, most clinicians agree that it *is not* censure, fault finding, or motivating by threats, guilt, or moralizing. These are usually abundantly available in your patients' daily lives. If change is to come about as a result of your care and rapport, you'll have to provide something altogether different.

Accepting people as they are is most difficult when it is most important. Dealing with patients is pleasant enough most of the time, but sooner or later you'll be involved with someone who has committed an offense that goes against everything you believe in. How will you deal with a parent who has burned an infant with lighted cigarettes and immersion in scalding bath water? Or less extreme, what about the person who comes to your office drunk, or the patient with diabetes who regularly fails to take insulin and overeats until diabetic acidosis results? These are the patients who test our professionalism.

Your feelings and actions in situations like these will be influenced by your own life experiences and your personal values. Sometimes you may feel good about how you handle yourself, and other times not so pleased. There are no absolute principles to guide you in each situation. One spokesman, the psychologist Carl Rogers, has focused attention on the concept of "unqualified positive regard." He writes in *Becoming a Real Person* (1961):

> ...I find that the more acceptance and liking I feel toward this individual, the more I will be creating a relationship which he can use. By acceptance I mean a warm regard for him as a person of unconditional self-worth—of value no matter what his condition, his behavior, or his feelings.

Another way of expressing the same thing is the dictum, "Separate the sin from the sinner: hate the sin but not the sinner."

□ RESPONSIBILITY

Accepting responsibility for what you do, or don't do, is difficult in any setting, and particularly when it involves responsibility for others. "The buck stops here," was Harry Truman's way of describing the presidency; the same is true in medical practice. Many decisions have to be made on the basis of uncertain information, without a lot of time for study or consultation. The responsibility comes with the job (and is one reason society is willing to pay physicians on a premium scale). Taking responsibility does not mean you guarantee success, only that you have a plan of action and that the patient knows to whom to turn for help, information, or just sharing a concern.

One of the unfortunate side-effects of medical specialization is the diffusion of responsibility, or its evaporation altogether. No one at all may be in charge (Carmichael, 1986).

The administrator of a large multispecialty medical group developed back pain that proved to be the first symptom of a cancer of the prostate. He was cared for by physicians in the group, all of whom were fond of him and wanted to do everything possible for what they knew would be a losing battle. No one, however, was in charge of his care, and no one realized the need to coordinate the efforts of the urologist, the radiotherapist, the orthopedist, and the chemo-therapist. Each provided excellent specialty care, but no one took responsibility for the whole person. Unconsciously, no one wanted the responsibility. When complications developed, the patient was passed from one doctor to the next. The patient was literally alone amid all the fine talents of his group. He would have felt better if he could have complained to someone, but his friendship with the staff made that impossible, and really ill patients rarely have the courage to criticize those on whom they depend. He wasn't conscious of these complicating social factors or of feeling abandoned; he just became deeply depressed. His depression seemed natural enough to others, considering his condition; no one appreciated the true reason.

Perhaps this section should have been the first one, for without a patient and a responsible clinician coming together, rapport is neither good or bad—it doesn't exist.

□ MONEY

Money may seem out of place in a chapter dealing with such lofty concerns as honesty, responsibility, and respect. But money is an intermediary, a measure of services, and one tangible expression of a clinician's motivation. The medical profession has a reputation, deserved or not, of being preoccupied with income.

While in medical school you will not deal directly with financial aspects of care, but, like other hidden agendas, they exert their influence. A patient who receives a staggering medical bill, even if partially or entirely covered by insurance, may feel exploited by those providing care, you included. Some patients look at an itemized bill and wonder whether all the services were really needed. They notice with mistrust cryptic abbreviations like PFT (pulmonary function test) or LHF (laboratory handling fee). While on your clerkship, get a copy of your patient's daily ledger to appreciate the financial aspects of care. Insensitivity to financial matters can seriously impair rapport. Smoldering resentment about charges and collection can ruin a relationship, and it sometimes triggers a malpractice suit that would otherwise never have occurred.

Types of practice, and differing methods of payment to physicians also influence rapport. The development of the Health Maintenance Organization (HMO) and Diagnosis Related Groups (DRG) fundamentally alters the financial relationship between patient and provider (Brody, 1985). In both instances, the physician or the organization employing the physician, gains income by providing fewer rather than more, services. The noted medical sociologist, David Mechanic (1985), comments

> As the payment of physicians shifts from a fee-for-service practice basis to alternative arrangements, we can anticipate some unwanted adjustments. Salaried physicians, as compared with those in fee-for-service practice, typically work fewer hours and, some would contend, less hard as well .... These changes inevitably bring challenges to the trust between patient and physician and possible conflict.

□ Rapport's Fulfillment: Care With Caring

□ CONTINUITY

Sometimes you do everything just right and still feel that things are not going well, that rapport isn't developing the way you would like it to. Don't be too hasty to blame yourself. Many people take their time in developing a trusting relationship with a clinician. It is the same way in relationships of all sorts. A certain amount of testing goes on. There have to be some shared experiences before acceptance develops. Some health care settings do not facilitate continuity. As a student or resident, you will shuttle from one service to the next, and lose contact with patients in the process.

There are no easy answers to staying in touch with your patients during your training, but it can be done. Hospitals publish a daily admission list, which you can scan for familiar names. Computers make possible automatic notification of readmission (Levinson, 1968). Occasional phone calls to patients no longer under your care are often appropriate and appreciated. Reviewing medical charts also provides valuable follow-up information.

When you know that you will be leaving a patient with whom you have an ongoing relationship, let the patient know far in advance. The patient needs time to find another health care provider. It is just as important to give the patient time to work through the separation. You may not realize just how important you are to a patient you see on a regular basis. Many will experience a real sense of loss when you leave. Well handled, however, the transition can be smooth, and you and your patient will separate with good feelings and memories (Lichstein, 1982).

☐ TRUST

Inherent in accepting responsibility for the patient's welfare is the concept of trust. People, when ill, are in no position to question everything you say and do, and few have the courage to ask (although patient education efforts are becoming an increasingly important aspect of comprehensive care). When a person becomes a patient, that person's welfare depends on the integrity of the caretaker. Where trust is violated, whether in small matters or large, the doctor-patient relationship loses its vitality.

☐ CARING

One of the essential qualities of the physician is interest in humanity, for the secret of the care of the patient is caring for the patient.

Dr. Francis Peabody (1923)

This statement could well serve as the maxim for establishing patient rapport. While continuing to emphasize "curing," good medicine also pays attention to its caring aspects. As a physician, although you will not always be able to cure a patient, you can always console. An unknown French author advised the medical profession "to cure sometimes, to relieve often, to comfort always." Rapport with your patients will minimize the sometimes frightening and dehumanizing experiences that increasingly occur in our highly structured, technology oriented medical system. Caring *for* a patient is more personal than the caring *of* the patient.

☐ RAPPORT IN OTHER CHAPTERS

Just as rapport pervades clinical practice, so will it reappear in this book. Here is a preview.

Rapport in your relationships with:

- ☐ Families.
- ☐ Children.
- ☐ Older people.
- ☐ Faculty.

☐ Staff.
☐ VIP's.

Practical matters affecting rapport:

☐ Time.
☐ Privacy.
☐ Keeping a confidence.
☐ Office staff interpersonal skills.
☐ Telephone medicine.
☐ Rapport and the "difficult patient."

☐ REFERENCES AND READINGS

Barsky AJ: Hidden reasons some patients visit doctors. Ann Intern Med 1981;94 (Part 1):492–498.
Beckman HB, Frankel RM: The effect of physician behavior on the collection of data. Ann Intern Med 1984;101:692–696.
Brody H: Ethical gatekeeping: the ongoing debate. J Fam Pract 1986;23:539–540.
Carmichael JK: Responsibility vs anonymity. J Fam Pract 1986;23:595–596.
Dunn JJ, Lee TH, Percelay JM, et al: Patient and house officer attitudes on physician attire and etiquette. JAMA 1987;257:65–68.
Engel GL: A life setting conducive to illness: the giving-up/given-up complex. Ann Intern Med 1968;69:293–304.
Golden A, Grayson M, Bartlett E, Barker LR: The doctor-patient relationship: communication and patient education. In Barker LR, Burton JR, Zieve PD: Principles of Ambulatory Medicine, ed 2. Baltimore, Williams & Wilkins, 1986, pp 30–41.
Griffith J: Getting physical with patients (letter). Medical Economics January 7, 1985, p 22.
Herwig TT: "I don't know." JAMA 1986;256:2348.
Korsch BM, Negrete V: Doctor-patient communication. Sci American 1972:227 (August):66–74.
Levinson D, Bartlett J, et al: Patient follow-up registry: An aid to clinical education. J Med Educ 1968;43:961–968.
Lichstein PR: The resident leaves the patient: another look at the doctor-patient relationship. Ann Intern Med 1982;96(Part 1):762–765.
Mechanic D: Sounding Board: Public perceptions of medicine. N Engl J Med 1985;312:181–183.
Older J: Teaching touch at medical school. JAMA 1984;252:931–933.
Peabody FW: The care of the patient. JAMA 1927;88:877–882. Reprinted as a Landmark Article in JAMA 1984;252:813–818. Also see Rabin PL, Rabin D: The care of the patient revisited. JAMA 1984;252:819–820.
Platt FW, McMath JC: Clinical hypocompetence: the interview. Ann Intern Med 1979;91:898–902.
Rakel RE, Levinson D: Establishing rapport. In Rakel RL (ed): Textbook of Family Practice, ed 3, Philadelphia, W. B. Saunders Company, 1984, pp 307–323.
Reiser DE, Rosen DH: Medicine as a Human Experience. Baltimore, University Park Press, 1984, p. 27.
Relman AS: The changing climate of medical practice. N Engl J Med 1987;316:333–334.
Rogers C: On Becoming A Person. Boston, Houghton Mifflin, 1961, p 33.
Waitzkin H: Doctor-patient communication: clinical implications of social scientific research. JAMA 1984;252:2441–2446.

UNIT **II**

PROBLEM-SOLVING

CHAPTER 5

DISEASE, ILLNESS, AND PROBLEM-SOLVING

The goal of the interview, physical examination, and laboratory testing is effective therapy. Effective treatment depends on identifying the disease to be treated. This chapter looks at the concept of disease and describes a diagnostic process that helps translate the patient's illness manifestations into a disease diagnosis.

☐ Concept of Disease

Disease is an elusive concept. *Disease* can be defined as an abnormality in structure or function. Several elements contribute to the disease process: *stress* or *injury* to a biological system plus *response* to the stress or injury.

A young woman falls asleep under a sun lamp, which remains on for 30 minutes. The ultraviolet rays damage the skin during the half-hour exposure, but she is unaware of the damage until 8–12 hours later, when the skin responds to the radiation injury with the inflammation of "sunburn"—redness, heat, swelling, and pain. The initial injury is silent; the disease is experienced by the patient as an illness due in part to the body's repair effects.

Pneumonia is a disease process initiated by a silent invasion of lung tissue by microbes. The invasion leads to a variety of not-so-silent defensive body responses: fever to augment metabolism, an out-pouring of white blood cells that engulf and destroy the bacterial invaders, and cough to expel expended masses of white blood cells (sputum). "Pneumonia" as experienced by the patient and observed by physicians is a manifestation of bodily defenses.

A young man, a somewhat passive and dependent only child who has lived at home throughout his college years, marries a woman who does not meet his parents' standards. Although the marriage gets off to a good start, he becomes significantly depressed. The unconscious stress (involving the mental system) is the loss of his parents' approval and caring. The depression is partly the mental system's attempt to restore the loss. The pain of depression atones for the unconscious guilt the patient feels for marrying against his parents' wishes, and the evident suffering elicits his parents' concern. Seen in the perspective of disease as defined above, the depression makes good sense in terms of repairing some of the effects of an important loss.

This concept of disease has three dimensions:
1. *Cause* (initiating and predisposing factors): *Why?*
2. *Location* (within a discrete organ or system): *Where?* (See Chapter 7 for the anatomical system used in this text.)
3. *Pathological process* (inflammation, neoplasm, obstruction, and so forth*): *What?*
Like all classifications, this one contains overlapping, inter-related processes and is not rigorously logical. Develop a classification that seems right to you. Pathological processes will be discussed in the next chapter.

Disease terminology should reflect this *cause-location-pathological process* concept. For example:

Viral hepatitis identifies cause to be a virus, the liver ("hepar") as the organ involved, and the pathological process as inflammation ("itis").

This definition of disease is expressed in a formula:

$$\text{Disease} = \text{Cause} + \text{Location} + \text{Pathological Process}$$
$$\text{Why?} \qquad \text{Where?} \qquad \text{What?}$$

This is not the pathologist's definition; it says little about the exact nature of the disease. It is a practical definition based on the information you obtain during the interview, physical examination, and laboratory testing. When you can make a statement about *cause, location,* and *pathological process,* you have defined disease in a way that uniquely identifies, or *diagnoses,* it. When you know the name of a disease, you are then able to determine appropriate therapy.

---

*Here is one classification of pathological processes:

□ Inflammation	□ Obstruction	□ Psychopathology
□ Neoplasia	□ Genetic	□ Nutritional
□ Degeneration	□ Toxic	□ Metabolic
□ Ischemia/Infarction	□ Allergy	□ Mechanical

The noun *diagnosis* is equivalent to naming the disease (The diagnosis is peptic ulcer disease). The verb *diagnose* refers to the problem-solving, or diagnostic process, leading to the disease identification ("We plan to diagnose your condition by X-ray studies.").

□ Diagnostic Process

The problem-solving method used to achieve a diagnosis is based on two steps:
1. Identifying the *causal* or *initiating* factors of the disease.
2. Analyzing the symptoms and signs by which the disease is expressed in the ill patient.
Cause is logically first, but, for reasons that will be explained later, in clinical practice the search for causes usually comes last in the interview sequence. Therefore, we will reorder the formula:

$$\text{Disease} = \text{Location} + \text{Pathological Process} + \text{Cause}$$
$$\text{Where?} \qquad \text{What?} \qquad \text{Why?}$$

□ Illness and Symptom Analysis

You, as a clinician, do not deal directly with disease (which you cannot observe in detail as the pathologist does) but with illness—the patient's *experience* of the injury and reaction to injury that make up disease as we have defined it. Illness is the experience of disease as manifested in symptoms and signs.

Symptoms are the subjective experience of disease. In the previous examples, the sunburn, cough, and depression are symptoms. Other symptoms are *nausea, blurred vision, palpitations, cramps.* Only the patient experiences symptoms; your understanding of the symptoms depends on what the patient tells you during the interview.

Signs are objective evidence of disease. A *blood pressure measurement*, a *rash*, a *mass in the abdomen* that you can feel, a *heart murmur* are all signs.

Symptom analysis is the chief focus of the diagnostic interview, and the first step in the *Problem-Centered* interview. Coming before the physical examination or laboratory testing, symptom analysis is the royal road to understanding the patient's disease *location* and *pathological* process.

□ Translating Illness Into Disease

Illness and *disease,* although related, are basically different. Patients think of themselves as having an "illness." Only after you analyze the illness can you talk about the patient's disease. The signs and symptoms of the patient's illness must be translated into a disease identification—a diagnosis.

The translation process must take into account four major factors:

1. Different diseases are expressed in similar illnesses.

2. A disease expresses itself differently at different stages of its natural course.

3. The same disease, at the same stage, is experienced differently by different persons.

4. Your qualities as interviewer and caretaker affect how patients report their illness.

☐ Different Disease, Similar Illness

There are thousands of diseases, but relatively few symptoms. The body has only a limited set of responses to a wide variety of disease-related factors.

Streptococcal pharyngitis and the pharyngitis associated with infectious mononucleosis both create an *illness* characterized by very similar symptoms and signs: sore throat, fever, general malaise, a whitish membrane on the tonsils and swollen lymph nodes. One condition, however, is caused by a bacteria, the other by a virus. Disease manifestations such as sore throat, fever, or swollen glands are usually *non-specific* that is, they commonly occur with a variety of diseases.

Both angina pectoris, a manifestation of potentially lethal coronary artery disease, and hiatal hernia, an uncomfortable but not serious condition of the diaphragm and stomach, share symptoms of retrosternal (behind the sternum) pressure or burning.

Hyperthyroidism (thyroid overactivity) and anxiety share a common pathway of sympathetic nervous system overactivity. Thus, an early stage of hyperthyroidism is often misdiagnosed as anxiety.

Even though different diseases are expressed in similar ways, some differences can be elicited by the history, physical examination, and various laboratory findings. Mononucleosis is associated with enlarged lymph nodes in many of the areas of the body, whereas the lymph node enlargement of streptococcal sore throat is limited to the upper neck. Angina and hiatal hernia share some symptoms but differ in others (their relationship to exertion, for example), and have altogether different findings on x-ray and electrocardiographic interpretation. Hyperthyroidism and anxiety are differentiated on the basis of psychological history and physical findings, and clearly separated by laboratory tests.

During the interview, the differences between similar illnesses are not always obvious. They are detected by attention to detail. The essence of the diagnostic challenge is discovering illness characteristics that distinguish one disease from another. Your role during the interview is to understand the illness both in its broad manifestations and in the differences that separate one condition from another.

□ Same Disease, Different Stage

Another barrier to accurate illness translation is that a disease is not the same from one moment to the next. A disease is an evolving process. It passes through a series of stages. Each stage has unique qualities that blend with those preceding and following. The early stage of appendicitis is different than appendicitis 24 or 36 hours later. Early rheumatoid arthritis is different in its overall manifestations than rheumatoid arthritis that has been present for years. You will never see two patients at exactly the same stage of the same disease.

□ Same Disease, Different Persons

Symptoms are *processed* by the patient's mental and neurological systems. This processing is similar to a stereo system in which the input from the radio receiver or record is amplified and shaped. A song may be kept to a low volume of background music or magnified to the ear-shattering level of a rock concert. Treble, bass, and equalizer controls offer infinite ways to modify the music reaching the listener. And quite apart from the musical input, the system itself creates some noise and distortion.

In the same way, patients vary widely in how they experience and report their illness. Some persons almost apologetically report symptoms that other persons describe in dramatic and urgent terms. Many variables influence the patient's history: cultural, social, psychological, and economic background all play a role. Some of these variables have been described in *Chapter 3: Seeking and Accepting Medical Care.*

In addition to personality variables are the differences in each person's biological response to stress and injury. No two individuals react the same way to the same underlying disease-causing agent. Immunity moderates or eliminates the body's response to microorganisms, and hence the illness. General health and age-related factors all modify the resulting illness.

One patient with viral bronchitis displays a slight cough and low grade fever. A patient with a prior history of asthma, upon exposure to the same virus, develops not only a cough and fever, but bronchospasm and associated wheezing. A third person, having developed immunity to the particular strain of infecting agent, displays no illness at all. Finally, someone who once nearly drowned may become highly anxious at the first sign of shortness of breath, however mild the disease process.

A fourth element—your influence on the patient—also enters into consideration. This factor will be discussed in *Chapter 20: Difficult Relationships.*

□ Problem-Solving

For the reasons listed above:
1. Symptoms shared by different diseases.
2. The different characteristics of the same disease at different stages.
3. The biological and psychological uniqueness of each person.

the interpretation of illness and its translation into a formal disease diagnosis is a challenging experience.

Clinical techniques and strategies are often successful in converting the data of illness into a useful disease definition, even at the initial stage of history-taking. The diagnostic process starts with two strategies of symptom interpretation:

□ Symptoms are *precisely characterized.*
□ Symptoms are *grouped into clusters.*

For the remainder of the book, only symptoms will be discussed, since signs are obtained through the physical examination. The boundary between symptoms and signs is a blurred one, however. In practice you often move between the two as you progress towards a diagnosis.

□ Characterizing Symptoms

Symptoms, *precisely described,* contain a world of information about the underlying disease. *Cough,* for example, has a generally understood meaning, but there are many different kinds of coughs. A cough may be deep, harsh, barking, loose, moist, dry, or whooping. A *detailed* description of the cough assists in identifying the disease causing the cough. The cough of pertussis (whooping cough) and of measles, for example, are so characteristic that an experienced physician can make a diagnosis as soon as the patient comes into the office. Patients with pneumonia characterize their cough differently than do patients with simple bronchitis. Similarly, the precise type of pain associated with myocardial infarction is different from that of pericarditis. There are always overlapping areas, however, and no clinician makes a judgment of the underlying disease based on the symptom description alone. But initial clues influence the direction of further questioning and examination. In Chapter 6 seven dimensions (*"The Sacred Seven"*) by which any symptom can be characterized will be detailed.

□ Clusters

You will not always deal with a single symptom or single sign. Even if a patient initially states a single complaint, other facets of the illness emerge as you interview the patient. As symptoms and signs are grouped, you may recognize characteristic patterns that correlate with specific diseases.

- □ *Sneezing, clear nasal discharge,* and *tearing eyes* taken together are consistent with hay fever.
- □ *Tremor, weight loss, hyperactivity,* and *diarrhea* all developing at about the same time are consistent with hyperthyroidism.
- □ *Nausea* and *vomiting, pain* starting in the mid-upper abdomen and then moving to the right lower quadrant, *fever,* and *constipation* are consistent with early appendicitis.

These clusters are more common in textbooks than in a real patients for the reasons already given. In fact, a patient with a "textbook" or "classic" case of some condition is the focus of great attention in teaching hospitals because such cases are so rare. There are some diseases, however, in which clusters of different manifestations are predictably present. Most of these conditions are hereditary and determined by a specific genetic abnormality. The questions of multiple symptoms and several co-existing diseases will be discussed in Chapter 10.

□ Causes of Disease

After symptom analysis to establish the *Where?* and the *What?* in the formula

$$\text{Disease} = \underset{\text{Where?}}{\text{Location}} + \underset{\text{What?}}{\text{Pathological Process}} + \underset{\text{Why?}}{\text{Cause}}$$

comes the search for *cause,* or *Why?* Let's look at some simple clinical examples in which the cause seems obvious.

A 31-year-old man who is unaccustomed to heavy work is repairing the foundation of his house. While lifting a 90-pound sack of cement he suddenly develops low back pain.

A 49-year-old man has had peptic ulcer disease, diagnosed by x-ray, for 12 years. He regularly develops his symptoms in the fall of the year. One day in September he develops an attack of upper abdominal pain.

A 37-year-old man develops chest pain while practicing for a marathon run. Both parents died in their 30's of coronary artery disease.

A 52-year-old woman develops chest pain and a continuing cough over the past six months. She has smoked three packs of cigarettes a day for the last 25 years.

A 25-year-old woman develops diarrhea shortly after returning from a trip to Mexico. She had visited a region in which amoebiasis was endemic, and during her visit she was careless about where and what she ate.

These examples represent clinical histories from which a reasonable diagnosis is established on the basis of "probable cause" of preceding events. Information of this sort—*risk factors*—traditionally is derived from the sections of the medical history entitled *Past Medical History, Family Medical History, Personal and Social History.* The uses of this kind of information, as well as some of important limitations, are described in detail in *Chapters 8: Risk Factors in Diagnosis and Treatment.*

As with the other concepts used in discussing disease, the definition of *cause* is greatly simplified. The "cause" or etiology of any disease, when studied in detail, turns out to be a complex, dynamic interaction of many factors. The streptococcal organism, while necessary for the development of streptococcal sore throat, is only one factor in the disease's development. Not everyone exposed to the organism becomes ill—host and environmental factors enter into the disease-producing equation. Your course in pathology will discuss many of these complexities and help you develop your own concept of disease. For now, however, a simplified idea of cause will be enough for you to get started in your problem-solving skills.

☐ Additional Comments About Disease

Localization of disease is something of a fiction. While some diseases, such as appendicitis, are localized, other diseases are multi-system. That one area is more symptomatic than another does not always reflect a significant localization of the basic disease. Rheumatoid arthritis, for example, often involves the skin, eyes, blood vessels and nerves as well as the joints. And the frequent urination occurring in diabetes reflects the high blood sugar level, which is a secondary manifestation of more basic dysfunctions affecting several metabolic systems.

Another aspect of the localization concept is that the *symptomatic* disease may be only a manifestation of some more remote but silent disorder. For example, a man who develops severe back pain may have a metastasis in his lumbar vertebra from prostatic cancer which was not in itself symptomatic. Shortness of breath may be the first manifestation of silent hypertension that, after months or years, has finally caused the heart to fail and fluid congestion in the lungs. Black stool, a sign of blood in the feces, may not indicate gastrointestinal bleeding but rather a slow but persistent posterior nosebleed from which the patient is swallowing the blood. Usually starting with the symptomatic condition allows you to trace back to the underlying but non-symptomatic disease.

Some diseases result from an exaggerated, deleterious reaction to stress—allergic conditions for example. Other diseases—many cancers and chronic diseases, for example—elicit so little body reaction that they are "silent" for tragically long periods. The reaction to injury of emphysema—a cough or mild shortness of breath, for example—is initially of little concern to most people, although it is a warning of worse things to come. *Health Promotion*, discussed in *Unit III*, specifically searches for silent conditions and seemly minor problems.

Not all stresses result in illness. Life is a continuing, dynamic and often silent process of adaptation to stresses of all types. When the process of adaptation exceeds a certain level, symptoms develop. Similarly, the distinction between stress and injury is blurred.

Some disease manifestations can be both signs and symptoms. The patient reports the *symptom*, "Feeling feverish"; you measure the *sign* of body temperature. A patient subjectively reports the symptom "Irregular heart beat"; "palpitations" or "skipped beats"; you objectively feel the sign of an irregular pulse and record the rhythm on an electrocardiogram.

Medical terminology is a confusing blend of precise and not-so-precise terminology. Few diseases are named in the rational "cause-location-process" format of *viral hepatitis:*

Carcinoma of the pancreas defines location and process, but says nothing about cause, which is not known.

Diabetes mellitus (literally, "the flowing through of honey") simply describes one clinical feature of a systemic disease of uncertain pathology and cause.

Paget's disease says nothing at all beyond the fact that there exists a condition initially described by Dr. Paget. In fact, there are two Paget's diseases, one affecting bone and one affecting skin, indicating how imprecise this terminology is.

Cliches and medical jargon are so important in our thinking and communicating that we risk dealing with words rather than people. Words are not *equivalent* to the things they represent, but medical terms sometimes take on a life of their own. Think about what words *refer to*, rather than the words themselves.

Not all problem-solving steps are understood; even master diagnosticians cannot tell exactly how they achieve their results (Elstein, 1978). If the process were fully understood and entirely rational, a computer could do it. Computer scientists are trying, but they are a long way from their goal, as discussed in *Chapter 30: Computers.*

☐ REFERENCES AND READINGS

Elstein AS, Shulman LS, Sprafka SA: Medical Problem-Solving: An Analysis of Clinical Reasoning. Cambridge, MA, Harvard University Press, 1978.
Feinstein A: Clinical Judgment. Baltimore, Williams and Wilkins, 1967.

CHAPTER 6

SYMPTOM ANALYSIS

□ SYMPTOMS AND DISEASE

Patients seek care because of *symptoms* (subjective awareness of an unaccustomed body or mental state). Your task is to translate these symptoms, along with information about risk factors, into a *diagnosis*—naming or identifying the specific disease that underlies the patient's illness. Disease has been defined in terms of three factors:

1. Location (Where?).
2. Pathological Process (What?).
3. Cause (Why?).

and expressed as a simple formula:

$$\text{Disease} = \text{Location} + \text{Pathological Process} + \text{Cause}$$
$$\phantom{\text{Disease} = }\text{Where?} \qquad \text{What?} \qquad \text{Why?}$$

The diagnostic aspects of a patient's problem are answered when you locate the source of the problem within an organ or system (Where?), make a judgment about the pathological process (What?), and identify a cause (Why?). This chapter explains how a clear understanding of the patient's symptoms gives you answers to the Where? and the What? The Why?, a more complicated question, is discussed in *Chapter 8: Risk Factors in Diagnosis and Treatment.*

The technique of symptom analysis is straightforward. You start with the term the patient uses to describe a symptom and refine it to a set of precise dimensions, characteristics, or parameters.

The words patients use to describe their symptoms are variable; sometimes the terms are vague and general, or they may reflect the patient's education or locale. What one person describes as a "pain" someone else describes as a

49

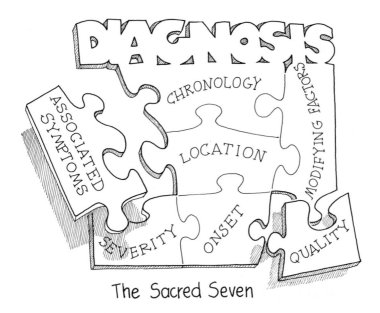

The Sacred Seven

"hurting sensation." A patient complaining of "stomach trouble" might mean diffuse discomfort anywhere in the abdomen, not just overlying the anatomical stomach in the upper abdomen. "Arthritis," or "nervous," or "indigestion," or "tired all the time" are other symptoms that require refinement before you can translate them into *organ/system* location and *pathological process.* Textbooks describe the pain of a heart attack as "pressure" or "crushing," but patients commonly report the sensation as a "burning." Jim Lehrer, noted TV journalist of the MacNeil Lehrer Nightly News Report, described his heart attack as "A dry tightness—like sand."

☐ THE *SACRED SEVEN*

The number of ways to look at a symptom is arbitrary. The approach used in this book defines *seven* dimensions that provide the information needed for a careful symptom analysis. (In fact, seven is so useful that we'll refer to the seven dimensions of a symptom as the *Sacred Seven.* In ancient times, seven was considered to have magical qualities—maybe the old-timers knew more about disease than we give them credit for.) These are the *Sacred Seven,* using the symptom of *pain* as an illustration.

1. **Location/Radiation:** In what place or area of the body does the patient feel the pain? In addition to the major focus, does it radiate, travel, or appear in other areas? Many symptoms are experienced in body areas overlying or near the diseased organ. Your knowledge of gross anatomy

will make clear those relationships. Some symptoms, however, are felt in unexpected areas. Pains appearing in atypical locations, referred pains, are discussed in detail at the end of the chapter. Since *organ/system* location (an element of disease definition), and *location/radiation* experienced by the patient are often similar, the term location is used in both contexts. As is noted below, however, there are some exceptions, so be sure you understand the two ways the term *location* is used.

2. **Chronology/Timing:** The duration of illness since onset; within the total duration are there daily, weekly, monthly, or seasonal patterns? How does the illness change over time?

3. **Quality:** What is the symptom "like?" What is its character—sharp, dull, burning, prickly, achy?

4. **Severity:** How intense? How extensive? How much? How "bad"? How does the symptom limit activity?

5. **Setting** or **Onset:** What was the patient doing when the illness started? Under what circumstances was the onset? Are there predictable events prior to the recurrence of the same symptom (as contrasted with events that worsen a symptom once it has started). Was the patient entirely well prior to the onset? (Sometimes the patient has been ill for months before some major or dramatic symptom occurs that results in getting medical attention. For example, a patient with a slowly growing brain tumor may ignore mild headaches for months and seek help only after a convulsion occurs.)

6. **Modifying Factors:** What makes the symptom better or worse? What has the patient tried to relieve it?

7. **Associated Symptoms:** What other symptoms accompany the chief or most prominent complaint?

Each of these dimensions contains information that helps you to define the *organ/system* disease location and the pathological process. Here is a case illustrating the reasoning involved in translating the seven dimensions of a patient's symptom into an *organ/system* and *pathological process* definition. Consider a 45-year-old man who has a pain "behind the breastbone" (retrosternal pain) with some radiation to the left side of the neck.

1. Among the organs or systems that create pain in this location are the heart, the respiratory system, and the upper gastrointestinal system (esophagus and stomach). (Other common organ/system locations include the rib cage (musculoskeletal system), the skin overlying the chest, and the mental system, but for the purposes of this example we will not consider these.) Symptom location, while suggesting some organs or systems, all but excludes others. The kidneys, for example, because of their innervation, do not refer pain to the retrosternal area.

2. If in questioning about chronology/timing you learn that the patient has

had this symptom "off-and-on" for 10 years, a malignant neoplasm as a pathological process is virtually excluded, since such tumors grow rapidly and continuously. If the pain is of only a few hours or days duration, almost any type of the many kinds of pathology involving the cardiovascular or respiratory systems is possible.

3. The pain's quality, if described as "burning," suggests esophageal or stomach irritation (chemical inflammation) from acid. This dimension, however, is not very specific. Some patients with bronchial inflammation, or with coronary artery disease, describe their experience as a "burning."

4. If the pain's severity is such that the patient has to stop all activity when the pain develops, an extensive pathological process (extensive heart disease or severe inflammation) is suggested. Again, the great variability in how different persons experience similar diseases makes this dimension difficult to interpret, but always worth asking about.

5. If the onset of the pain was in a setting of severe physical exertion, a cardiac or respiratory condition is more likely than a gastrointestinal one.

6. If modifying factors include the fact that deep breathing or coughing aggravates the symptom, and shallow breathing or inhaling moist vapor produces temporary relief, the respiratory tract is once again suggested as the disease site. If, on the other hand, inhaling soothing vapors produces little or no change in the symptom, but heavy exertion aggravates it and rest relieves it, the heart is the more likely primary disease site. Worsening of the pain when eating certain foods, and relief of pain with antacids is consistent with a gastrointestinal condition.

□ THE SEVENTH DIMENSION

The seventh dimension, *associated symptoms*, is particularly valuable in the diagnostic process, but is not easy for a beginning clinician to understand. The assumption is made that if a particular *organ/system* is the site of the disease, several other less prominent symptoms, in addition to the major complaint (in this example, *pain*) from the same organ or system are likely to be present. If, for example, in addition to the chest pain, the patient, when asked, recalls some difficulty with swallowing, unaccustomed belching, an episode of vomiting and mild diarrhea, then a disorder somewhere in the gastrointestinal system is suggested. The fact that these symptoms were not mentioned initially reflects the fact that they are not particularly bothersome and, in the patient's mind not significant. On the other hand, if none of these gastrointestinal symptoms are present, but the chest pain is accompanied with palpitations or irregular heart beat, shortness of breath with exertion, orthopnea (difficulty breathing when lying down), ankle swelling (edema), all a part of the cardiovascular system *Review of Systems* (to be discussed in the next chapter), this information tends to "rule out" the gastrointestinal system and "rule in" the cardiovascular system as the locale of the disease.

□ REFERRED PAINS

The neurological mechanism underlying unusual pain patterns, called *referred* pains, can usually be explained on the basis of embryological shifts in organ position. The sensory nerve fibers that supply the heart also mix their signals with afferent nerves from the upper thorax, arms, neck (T1–T4), and the face. The lower intercostal nerves, which transmit sensation from the pleura overlying the right lower lobe of the lung (T10–T11), also supply the upper abdomen. The under surface of the diaphragm, innervated by the phrenic nerve arising at the level of C4, is irritated by an injured spleen. Common referred pain patterns are:

Coronary artery disease is experienced in the retrosternal area, somewhat to the right of the heart's anatomical location, but also in the neck, either shoulder, either arm (the left most often), or in the jaw or face.

Inflammation of the lower lobe of the right lung may be reported by the patient as pain in the right upper quadrant of the abdomen.

An injured spleen is often associated with left shoulder pain.

A kidney stone in the ureter sends its pain to the testicle or labia.

For a discussion of referred pain see Engel (1983).

□ PATHOLOGICAL PROCESS

Determining what *pathological process* is present from symptom analysis is more difficult than is identifying disease location; structures are easier to define than functions. Several kinds of information will help you.

When you have identified the probable *organ/system* of a disease process, you often narrow the range of probable pathological processes, since each organ/system is more prone to certain diseases than others. For example, the heart is often diseased as a result of vascular ischemia/infarction, but only infrequently by neoplasms. The likely disease process is also limited to some extent by age of the patient. For example, infection frequently affects the prostate gland of younger men, whereas cancer predominates in older men.

The symptom characteristics (the first six dimensions of the *Sacred Seven*) of some pathological processes are fairly reliable.

Some pathological processes form clusters of symptoms that are reflected in the "associated symptoms" (the seventh dimension of the *Sacred Seven*).

In the previous chapter, the following classification of pathological processes was presented:

□ Inflammation.   □ Toxic.
□ Neoplasia.   □ Allergy.
□ Degeneration.   □ Psychopathology.
□ Ischemia/Infarction.   □ Nutritional.
□ Obstruction.   □ Metabolic.
□ Genetic.   □ Mechanical.

Not all of these processes have reliable correlates in the *Sacred Seven*. Part of the problem is that current disease classifications such this one are not internally consistent; they mix structural, functional, and etiological entities. Perhaps a better system of classification will produce more clinical uniformity. When you have studied pathology, the whole question will be clearer, but even without a knowledge of pathology the above guidelines will help you formulate a preliminary diagnosis. Remember that, in addition to the clinical history, you will obtain diagnostic information from the physical examination and laboratory testing.

Here are pathological processes that do have fairly dependable clinical manifestations or clusters:

Inflammation: fever, redness, swelling, pain.

Neoplasia (malignant or cancerous): unexplained weight loss, low-grade fever, masses which are often non-tender, unexplained bleeding, lesions that fail to heal, persisting alteration in any body function (for example, persisting and worsening difficulty in swallowing) that is progressive and not followed by long periods of activity or inactivity. (Except for enlarging masses, *benign neoplasms* lack these characteristics.)

Degeneration: gradual deterioration in structure and function, often over a period of years, for example, the gradual loss of the shiny, extremely smooth cartilage of joints affected by degenerative arthritis (osteoarthritis).

Ischemia/Infarction (partial or complete cessation of blood supply to a part of the body): dysfunction in relation to activity (such as exercise or eating) relieved by cessation of the activity; sudden dysfunction to a region of the body (such as neurological deficits immediately after a stroke), or obvious circulatory impairment of limbs (cold, pale, atrophic).

Obstruction: "colicky" pain—rhythmic, painful contractions associated with strong peristaltic smooth muscle contraction, repeated regularly every few minutes. Examples include uterine contractions of labor, contractions of a ureter obstructed by an entrapped kidney stone, or bowel contractions with bowel obstruction.

Genetic: multi-organ, multisystem structural and/or functional disorders often in several family members.

Allergy: itching, sneezing, hives, tearing, clear nasal discharge, periodicity especially in relation to timing patterns like seasons or specific environmental settings.

Psychopathology: alterations of thoughts, emotions, or behavior.

Mechanical: visible or palpable disruptions or physical alterations, such as laceration or bone fracture in relation to physical stresses.

Nutritional and *metabolic* diseases cover a wide spectrum with few unifying characteristics.

There are many exceptions to these characteristics. Specific cancers, for example, vary greatly in their clinical manifestations, especially in the early stages. Context also must be considered: in early appendicitis, neither swelling nor redness of the appendix can be detected by abdominal examination (although they are apparent at surgery).

As you interview, detailed information about the patient's symptom begins to suggest *probable* organ/system and pathological process involvement. Symptoms are, to a greater or lesser degree, not specific to just one organ/system or one pathological process. But as you question the patient, the weight of evidence begins to favor one possibility more than another. The diagnostic process is one of sorting out the evidence and assigning each symptom to the *organ/system* affected and the pathological process most likely present.

□ EXAMPLES OF THE *SACRED SEVEN*

Analyzing a symptom such as pain in terms of the seven dimensions is clear-cut. But what about a non-pain symptom such as bleeding—how can it be analyzed in the same framework? Here, in outline form, is the analysis of the symptom of "nosebleed" in a 40-year-old woman.

1. **Location/Radiation:** Is the bleeding anterior, coming out of the nares, or posterior, draining into the pharynx? Is there bleeding elsewhere (equivalent to *radiation*) such as gums, vagina, rectum, in the urine?

2. **Chronology:** Total duration since onset; within the total duration are there daily, weekly, monthly (relation to menses), or seasonal patterns?

3. **Quality:** What is the blood "like"? What is the color (bright red is consistent with arterial bleeding, dark red suggests a venous source)? Are there clots (indicating the clotting mechanism is functioning normally)?

4. **Severity:** How much bleeding (get a measure if possible, such as a teaspoonful, a cupful, used up a box of blood-soaked tissues or saturated a hand towel)?

5. **Setting** or **Onset:** What was the patient doing? Under what circumstances was the onset? Are there predictable events prior to the recurrence of the same symptom? Was the patient entirely well prior to the onset? (A

nosebleed might be the first dramatic event of a condition such as leukemia, which in the early stages may be associated only with fatigue or "just not feeling well.")

6. **Modifying Factors:** What makes the symptom better or worse? What has the patient tried to relieve it? Patients try all sorts of home remedies for nosebleeds, including a few like packing the nose with materials that lead to complications or make the condition worse.

7. **Associated Symptoms:** What other symptoms accompany the chief or most prominent complaint? The questions asked here depend on which organ/system of the body you decide to evaluate. Two reasonable organ/system possibilities, and their accompanying symptoms, are listed.

□ Nose and Sinuses: Stuffy nose, nasal discharge, head pain, unusual odors, nasal congestion.
□ Hematologic (Blood Forming): Bruising, weakness, pounding heart, trouble stopping bleeding from minor cuts, swollen glands.

These questions are the *Review of Systems* (ROS) for the two organs/systems selected. The ROS, and its usefulness in the problem-centered interview, is described in *Chapter 7: Review of Systems*. In this example, all of the *Sacred Seven* dimensions apply, with slight modification, to the analysis of the symptom of nosebleed.

□ ANALYSIS OF DIARRHEA AS A SYMPTOM

For some symptoms, one or more of the seven dimensions can be omitted. Common sense will guide you. For example, with "diarrhea," *location* is obvious (although "rectal bleeding" may not be: women may be unable to distinguish bleeding from the rectum from vaginal bleeding). All the other dimensions have valuable information and should not be omitted.

2. **Chronology/timing:** "Every 10 minutes." "Twice a day."

3. **Quality:** "Watery." "Full of blood." "Soft."

4. **Severity:** "Would guess about a pint of fluid every time." "Not a lot, maybe a cupful."

5. **Onset/setting:** "Right after I came back from Mexico."

6. **Modifying factors:** "If I eat anything solid, I get it." "Pepto-Bismol stops it for a couple of hours."

7. **Associated symptoms:** The *Gastrointestinal ROS*, also the *Systemic ROS* for symptoms like fever, weight loss.

□ ANALYSIS OF MULTIPLE SYMPTOMS

It is nice when patients complain of just one clear-cut symptom. In reality, they may present you with several symptoms at the very beginning of the interview. Applying the *Sacred Seven* to three of four symptoms will soon exhaust you and your patient. Fortunately, this is rarely necessary. Three strategies help you out.

1. Look for the most specific of the patient's symptoms, and focus on that one. For example, a patient may complain of fever, chills, fatigue and ear ache. Of these four symptoms, the ear ache is the most specific and the place to start.

2. Determining chronology. Which symptom came first? What has been the course of symptoms? When was the patient last entirely well? The answers may help you to identify a key symptom.

3. If a set of symptoms are all specific, involving separate organs, the patient may have a true *syndrome* (a set of disease manifestations that occur together). Syndromes involve multiple systems. They may be genetic diseases, multisystem diseases such as rheumatoid arthritis or diabetes mellitus, or a primary disease with secondary complications such as leukemia complicated by severe mouth inflammation.

Recognizing these conditions is partly a matter of pattern recognition—you, or someone you consult, have seen it before. There are no simple answers, but a variety of diagnostic methods are discussed in *Chapter 10: Diagnostic Strategies.*

□ WHERE NEXT?

Thus far, we have demonstrated how analysis of a symptom is a powerful diagnostic tool is helping identify the *Where?* and *What?* of the disease definition

$$\text{Disease} = \text{Location} + \text{Pathological Process} + \text{Cause}$$
$$\text{Where?} \qquad\qquad \text{What?} \qquad\qquad \text{Why?}$$

In *Chapter 8* we'll look at the kind of help analysis of *risk factors* provides in identifying causes. Please note one important feature of the analytic process being described. The emphasis thus far has been on identifying the *organ* or *system*, not on leaping to the name of the disease. This is quite different from the diagnostic method of experienced physicians: listening to the history and then proposing a specific disease such as pneumonia or colitis. Sometimes this approach works, sometimes not. If the correct disease diagnosis is missed, then it is back to the beginning, trying to match the patient's symptoms with another disease. When just beginning your diagnostic skill development, it is sounder to "think organ/system." This intermediate stage between illness and disease is a powerful help in knowing what to do next in the further evaluation of the patient. For example, to evaluate a patient with chest pain, a "GI Workup" or a "Heart Workup" is straightforward, whereas trying to make a specific diagnosis of every gastrointestinal or cardiovascular disease is impossible. See *Chapter 10: Diagnostic Strategies* for other aspects of the diagnostic process.

□ REFERENCE

Engel GL: Pain. *In* Blacklow RS (ed): MacBryde's Signs and Symptoms, ed 6. Philadelphia, JB Lippincott, 1983, Ch 3.

CHAPTER 7

REVIEW OF SYSTEMS

ROS, System/Symptom Review

☐ The ROS and the *Sacred Seven*

This chapter carries further the organ/system approach towards diagnosis, which starts with the patient's symptoms and identifies one or several possible organs or systems as the probable source of the patient's illness. In the last chapter you saw how a selective Review of Systems fulfilled the objectives of the seventh dimension, associated symptoms, in analyzing the symptom of chest pain in a 45-year-old man. Two factors are involved:

1. First, the assumption is made that if a particular organ/system is the site of the disease, several other less prominent symptoms, in addition to the major complaint, such as pain, are likely to be present. The presence or absence of a symptom tends to "rule out" or "rule in" the organ/system of the body with which the symptom is associated.

2. A second part of the *associated symptoms* questioning focuses on symptoms that reflect the pathological process, such as cancer, inflammation, obstruction, allergy, or metabolic imbalance.

The ROS enables you to examine organs or systems, not with your hands or with x-rays, but with words. Symptom characteristics, the *Sacred Seven*, rarely do more than narrow the problem to two or three organs or systems. The selective ROS then indicates which of the systems is more likely to be involved.

Another case illustrates these principles and the valuable role the selective ROS plays in clinical reasoning. Consider a 27-year-old woman who comes to

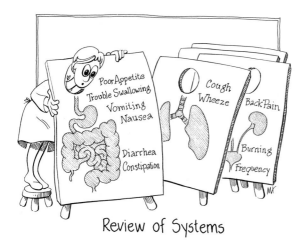

Review of Systems

you because of abdominal pain, nausea, and low-grade fever. As you analyze the symptom of the pain, you learn the following:

1. **Location:** Right lower quadrant of the abdomen. Pain does not radiate (go to other areas of the body).

2. **Chronology:** Pain present for 24 hours, more or less continuously.

3. **Quality:** Dull ache.

4. **Severity:** Mild discomfort, but enough that she did not go to work.

5. **Onset:** Gradual, no unusual activities preceded the illness.

6. **Modifying Factors:** Nothing seems to make the pain better; jarring movements, such as going over a bump in the car on the way to the clinic or pressing on the lower abdomen, causes increase in pain.

7. **Associated Symptoms:** At this point your thinking may go something like this: The fever and abdominal tenderness are consistent with inflammation, and infection is the most common (but not only) source of inflammation in this area of the body. The more difficult question is localization of the disease process. The right lower quadrant of the body is occupied by the gastrointestinal system (ileum, appendix, first portion of the large bowel), and the genitourinary system (ureters and bladder, ovaries, Fallopian tubes). A disorder of either system could create the type of pain the patient reports. Can additional questioning further localize the site of her disease? To complete the *Sacred Seven* you will have to ask about the Associated Symptoms (a selective ROS). You therefore inquire about the symptoms associated with disorders of the *gastrointestinal* and *genitourinary* systems. We'll list

Gastrointestinal System

Symptoms	Presence
Weight Change	No
Poor Appetite	Yes, Since Onset
Indigestion	Yes, Since Onset
Trouble Swallowing	No
Belching	No
Nausea	No
Vomiting	No
Vomiting Blood	No
Gas	No
Cramps	Yes, Since Onset
Change in Bowel Habits	Yes, Since Onset
Diarrhea	No
Constipation	Yes, Since Onset
Bleeding From Rectum	No
Hemorrhoids	No
Abdominal Swelling	No
Other	No

Genitourinary System

Urinary Symptoms	Presence
Painful Urination	No
Bloody or Cloudy Urine	No
Frequent Urination	No
Trouble Starting, Stopping, or Holding Urine	No
Other	No

Genital Symptoms (Female)	Presence
Last Menstrual Period (LMP)	Two Months Ago
Vaginal Bleeding	Spotting in Past Week
Menstrual Pain or Cramps	Yes
Vaginal Discharge	Yes
Change in Menstrual Pattern	Yes
Absent Periods	Missed Last Period
Hot Flashes	No
"Change of Life"/Menopause	No
Vaginal Itching	No
Other	No

the relevant ROS symptoms and the patient's answers as to whether any of these symptoms are present.

Looking over the three sets of symptoms, the cluster of positive symptoms related to the genital system suggests something is going on there. The absence of any urinary symptoms tends to eliminate that system as the source of the patient's disease. The gastrointestinal symptoms, especially the cramps and recent onset of constipation, are consistent with some gastrointestinal disease. Some of these gastrointestinal symptoms, especially the nausea and indigestion, are relatively nonspecific and accompany illnesses of many body systems.

The result of the symptom analysis suggests, but does not prove, that the patient's illness is located in the genital organs, although the gastrointestinal system cannot be excluded. This is about as far as a careful symptom analysis can take you. But you are now in a far better position to continue your history taking, physical examination, and laboratory testing than before. The selective ROS, particularly, has suggested the probable disease location. By "checking out" each system you think is involved in a patient's disease, you have moved closer to achieving an organ/system location—the Where? of the formula

$$\text{Disease} = \text{Location} + \text{Pathological Process} + \text{Cause}$$
$$\text{Where?} \qquad \text{What?} \qquad \text{Why?}$$

Similar reasoning was used in the two cases discussed in the previous chapter: the 45-year-old man with chest pain and the 40-year-old woman with a nosebleed.

The function of the ROS must be understood in terms of the goals of the problem-centered interview. Since you are trying to diagnose an illness, you limit your inquiry to the organs/systems most likely to be involved. For example, the ROS of the eyes was not included in the interview of either the man with the chest pain or the woman with bleeding discussed in *Chapter 6: Symptom Analysis*. There are well over 150 symptoms questions in a complete ROS; asking all of them in a brief problem-centered interview will frustrate both you and the patient. More importantly, only a few are relevant to any one clinical problem.

☐ Specific Symptoms

The ROS contains both specific and nonspecific symptoms. A specific symptom is one which often (not always) accompanies a disease of one organ or system; its presence helps to locate a disease. "Burning urination" is such a symptom; it points to the genitourinary system as the site of disease. Most symptoms are not entirely specific to just one organ/system; they occur regularly with diseases of one system, and less often accompany diseases of other systems. Vomiting, for example, frequently occurs in gastrointestinal diseases, sometimes accompanies diseases of the middle ear, the respiratory tract, reproductive system, central nervous system, and mental system, and often accompanies severe pain or severe infection anywhere in the body.

☐ Nonspecific Symptoms

A nonspecific symptom occurs with a disease in any part of the body. Fever, for example, accompanies inflammatory disease regardless of location and occurs as well in noninflammatory conditions including cancer, disorders of the temperature-regulating center of the brain, and endocrine conditions.

Other nonspecific symptoms include fatigue, weight loss, poor appetite, and nausea. The listing of a symptom with one organ/system of the ROS, therefore, does not mean that the same symptom might not accompany disease of some other organ/system.

□ The ROS and the Health Promotion Interview

The ROS in the Health Promotion history is, in effect, the Present Health. Sometimes when asked, patients remember symptoms that they had not considered to be significant, but that you recognize as indicative of disease.

□ The ROS During The Physical Examination

The ROS need not always be done during the interview. Part or all of the ROS can be done during the physical examination. Sometimes "laying on hands" helps the patient recall symptoms that might otherwise not be mentioned.

□ Think Organs/Systems, Not Diseases

The strategy just described is based on an *organ/system approach* to diagnosis. Notice that nothing was said about the possible *diseases* that could account for the patient's illness. No attempt is made to go from the patient's description of the illness directly to a specific disease. It is nice if it can be done, but it is not a reliable diagnostic method, particularly when you are just beginning your clinical experience. Rather than say, after gathering the clinical data, "This sounds like appendicitis, or maybe pelvic inflammatory disease, or an ectopic pregnancy, or a kidney stone," you and your patients are far better off if you say, "This sound like a gastrointestinal problem, or maybe a genitourinary problem." As has been mentioned before, and will be mentioned again, jumping from the illness description directly to a prognosis is risky. The variability of disease in any one patient, discussed in *Chapter 5: Disease, Illness, and Problem-Solving,* leads even experienced clinicians into difficulty more often than they might admit when they try to go directly from symptoms to a specific disease.

The *Think Organs/System* approach has several virtues:

□ When just beginning your clinical career, your knowledge of diseases is limited. But as soon as you have had courses in anatomy and physiology you are well-equipped to understand a systems approach to illness.

□ There are only a handful of major body systems; there are thousands of individual diseases.

□ Once you have established that a patient's illness involves one or more organs/systems, the next diagnostic steps of *system-focused* physical examination and laboratory testing are straightforward. Attempting to confirm a specific disease, on the other hand, can be a complex undertaking.

□ Major Organs/Systems

Here is a classification of major organs/systems:

□ Skin.
□ Eyes.
□ Ears, Nose and Sinuses, Mouth and Throat.
□ Pulmonary.
□ Cardiovascular.
□ Digestive.
□ Genitourinary.
□ Hematologic.
□ Immune.
□ Endocrine.
□ Musculoskeletal.
□ Nervous.
□ Mental.

This is a simplified and somewhat arbitrary classification; others are possible. One person might call the liver/gallbladder a separate system, rather than a sub-division of the digestive system. Many organs functionally are a part of several systems. The pancreas, for example, is both a digestive and endocrine organ, and the ears, nose, and throat have respiratory functions. Any classification you are comfortable with will serve the purpose of helping you "think organs/systems." Diagnostic errors do not result from a faulty classification system, but from failing to view the patient's illness from the perspective of *several different* but possible systems.

A special comment is warranted regarding the *Mental System*. Many persons do not recognize such a system and view all mental phenomena as the result of neurological processes. At the biochemical level they may be correct, but at the level of person-to-person interaction the mental system, or mind, can be evaluated without a knowledge of the neural sciences. Thoughts, emotions, and behaviors with which we solve problems, express feelings, communicate, make plans, and test reality comprise the science of psychology, a field of knowledge with reliable scientific principles and terminology. The mental system participates in every illness and should be considered in every diagnostic and therapeutic problem. In some diagnostic problems involving puzzling bodily symptoms, a psychological conversion reaction may be the fundamental mechanism (Engel, 1983). Since conversion symptoms mimic with great precision bodily symptoms, patients with such problems are often put through extensive medical testing. Often unwise therapies, including exploratory surgery, are undertaken in the search for an "organic" cause. Thinking about the mental system in perplexing problem-solving situations will often be rewarding.

□ Interviewing Techniques and the ROS

The ROS is rarely appreciated or used to its full potential. It is sometimes called a time-consuming, unproductive "wastebasket," and skipped over as quickly as possible. This unglamorous reputation is undeserved. A lot depends on the interviewing technique employed. You will find the ROS a powerful analytic tool, *provided* you note a few details of interviewing technique that reduce the time needed to ask the ROS and at the same time increases its accuracy.

The first time-saver is to avoid asking if the patient has *ever* had a certain symptom. The ROS is intended to detect *current or recurrent symptoms,* and there is no point in directing the patient's attention to past symptoms that no longer are a part of an active medical problem. Furthermore, most of the symptoms of a standard ROS have been experienced as part of a minor illness by almost everyone at *some time* in their lives. Occasionally, it is true, some past symptom has relevance to the present illness; the technique to be presented shortly usually detects such symptoms.

To increase the yield of the ROS, ask the *entire* ROS for the systems you are checking. Rarely does a patient report more than a few of the symptoms associated with any one system. To pick and choose among the symptoms lessens your chances of discovering those that are present.

The simplest and most effective technique to both save time and increase the yield of the ROS is to simply *mention* the symptom wihout suggesting past or present. For example: "How are your lungs and breathing? cough? sputum? shortness of breath? wheezing? pain on breathing? coughing up blood?" If you do this with a very brief pause between each question, patients usually respond if the mentioned symptom is now or ever has been a significant problem. Notice in this example that the *first question was the broadest possible one.* For example, to quickly cover the urinary system, ask "How are your kidneys and urination?" before going on to specific symptoms. Another minor detail, but one which consumes a lot of time, is introducing each symptom with "Do you have . . ." or something similar. You may find yourself doing this without realizing it; listening to a tape recording of yourself interviewing will call it to your attention.

Exactly how to phrase a question depends on your patient's level of education and medical sophistication. You can usually estimate your patient's familiarity with medical terms and concepts within the first few minutes of the interview. Be cautious about using jargon. *Dyspnea* is shortness of breath; *nocturia* is urinating at night; *polydypsia* is thirst. If you carry over the medical terms you use with other professionals into the interview, you risk confusing your patients (who, however, might not speak up and say they don't understand; instead, they may just answer "No" to each symptom).

□ Review of Systems (ROS)

Skin Any skin problems? ... itching? sores? rashes? growths or lumps? temperature or color changes? hair or nail changes? dryness? other?

Eyes How are your eyes and vision? ... blurred vision? pain? redness? infection or redness? discharge? eye strain? double vision? watery eyes? blind spots? other?

Ears, Nose, Throat (ENT)

Ears How are your ears and hearing? ... drainage? runny ears? poor hearing? ringing noises? spinning sensation? other ... ?

Nose and sinuses How are your nose and sinuses? ... stuffy nose? discharge? bleeding? head pain? unusual odors? congestion? (frequent colds?) other ... ?

Mouth Any problems in your mouth? ... sores? bad taste? sore tongue? bad teeth? gum trouble? other ... ?

Throat/Neck Any problems with your throat or neck? ... Sore throat? hoarseness? masses? swelling? trouble swallowing? other ... ?

Pulmonary

Any problems with your lungs or breathing? ... cough? chest pain? sputum? bloody cough? wheezing? chest noises? shortness of breath? (last chest x-ray?) other ... ?

Cardiovascular

Heart How is your heart? ... chest pain? pressure, tightness, or heaviness? rapid or irregular heart beat? shortness of breath? cough? swelling of feet? trouble breathing when flat in bed? weakness on exertion? fatigue? dizziness or fainting? (high blood pressure or heart disease?) other ... ?

Vascular How is your circulation? ... cold hands or feet? swelling? leg cramps? (varicose veins, phlebitis?) other ... ?

Digestive System

Gastrointestinal How is your digestion? . . . poor appetite? weight change? indigestion? trouble swallowing? belching? nausea? vomiting? vomiting blood? gas? cramps? swelling or fullness of abdomen? change in bowel habits? diarrhea? constipation? bleeding from rectum? hemorrhoids? other . . . ?

Liver and Gallbladder Any liver or gallbladder problems? . . . jaundice (or yellow skin or eyes)? indigestion? dark urine? pale or white stools? pain in upper abdomen? sudden dislike of tobacco (if patient smokes)? (hepatitis?) other . . . ?

Genitourinary

Urinary Any problems with kidneys or urination? . . . painful urination? bloody or cloudy urine? frequent urination (how often)? trouble starting, stopping, or holding urine? (frequent urinary infections?) other . . . ?

Genital (Male) Any problems with your sex organs? . . . pus or "drip" from the penis? sores on the penis? painful or swollen testicles? (venereal diseases like syphilis or gonorrhea?) other . . . ?

Genital (Female) Pregnancies? . . . abortions or miscarriages? . . . any menstrual difficulties or problems with your sexual organs or function? . . . last menstrual period (LMP)? vaginal bleeding? menstrual pain or cramps? vaginal discharge? absent periods? hot flashes? change of life/menopause? change in menses? vaginal itching? (venereal diseases like syphilis or gonorrhea?) other . . . ?

Breasts Any problems with your breasts? . . . lumps? nipple discharge? bleeding? swelling? tenderness? pain? do breast self-examination? other . . . ?

Hematologic

Any blood problems? . . . bruising? weakness? unusual paleness? pounding heart? bleeding anywhere? swollen glands? (transfusions?) other . . . ?

Immune

Frequent infections? . . . hives? . . . allergic reactions to foods, medicines, pollens, dust, insect bites? other . . . ?

Endocrine

Any problems with your (endocrine) glands? . . . change in general appearance? feeling hot or feeling cold all the time? unusual weight gain or weight loss? loss of appetite? thirst? change in skin or body hair? frequent urination? fatigue? tremor? other . . . ?

Musculoskeletal

Any problem with bones, joints, or muscles? . . . arthritis? red, swollen, or painful joints? muscle pain or tenderness? stiffness? muscle cramps? weakness? neck or back pain? arm or leg pains? limitation of movement? other . . . ?

Nervous System

Central Nervous System Any problems with your nervous system? . . . headache? weakness of an arm or leg? numbness? "blackouts"? dizziness? fainting? convulsions (fits)? trouble speaking? trouble walking or with balance or coordination? clumsiness? difficulty controlling bladder or bowels? trouble thinking? failing memory? other . . . ?

Peripheral Nervous System Weakness? numbness? "pins and needles"? other . . . ?

Mental (Mind)

How are your emotions and state of mind? . . . worry? "nervous" tension? fear? irritability? blueness or depression? bad dreams? trouble sleeping? suicidal thoughts? sexual trouble? unreasonable fears? tiredness? memory trouble? crying? hopeless? drinking or drug problem? uncontrollable or frightening thoughts or behavior? feeling people are out to get you? (mental illness?) other . . . ?

Systemic (Not localized to one system)

Any general symptoms? . . . fever? weight change? nausea? fatigue? poor appetite? just not feeling well? general health? other . . . ?

A few questions, shown in parentheses, logically refer to past illnesses, but many physicians find it practical to include them in the ROS. You can decide otherwise. As long as you know why you are asking a question, the exact location in the interview is of secondary importance.

Note that each system review starts with a broad, open-ended question ("Any problems with . . . ?" or "How are . . . ?"). In this way you help the patient focus on the organ system and function to be covered. When you are under great time pressure and feel that a system is unlikely but you don't want to dismiss the possibility altogether, asking one broad question gives the patient a chance to contribute information.

The symptom "other," which appears in each set of symptoms, is the most important "symptom" of all. The ROS is made up of *words*. Symptoms are experiences. Patients describe their symptoms in a variety of ways. For example, diarrhea, loose bowels, runs, trots, miseries are just a few of the terms patients may use for the same symptom. If you ask only about "diarrhea," the answer will not be meaningful if your patient isn't familiar with that term. The "other" reminds you to be alert to terms that are meaningful to the patient, even though you may not use the terms yourself.

Memorize the ROS as well as you can so that you have a good working knowledge of it. The task really isn't as difficult as it may seem, since almost all of the symptoms on the list are those you have personally experienced at one time or another. For example, just about everyone has at some time had a mild gastrointestinal disorder, and with it came most of the symptoms listed on the GI System catalog. The same for a common respiratory disorder like bronchitis, with its catalog of symptoms of cough, sputum, some shortness of breath, and chest pain. Don't rely entirely on memory, however; keep the ROS on a 3×5 card as a reminder and memory jog.

Despite its exceptional usefulness in localizing disease, the *Review of Systems* has limitations. Many symptoms, like fainting, weakness, chest pains, or shortness of breath arise from several systems. Sometimes ambiguity creates confusion—for example, "Any problems with your nervous system?" may be misinterpreted by the patient as an inquiry about mental (psychological) function. Rephrasing a question, or giving an explanation or example when the patient seems uncertain about what you want to know, will resolve the difficulty.

□ REFERENCES

Engel GL: Conversion symptoms. *In* Blacklow RS (ed): MacBryde's Signs and Symptoms, ed 6. Philadelphia, JB Lippincott, 1983, Ch 30.
Ford CV, Polks DG: Conversion disorders: An overview. Psychosomatics 1985;26:371–372.

CHAPTER 8

RISK FACTORS IN DIAGNOSIS AND TREATMENT

☐ Risk Factors and Causes of Disease

The previous two chapters demonstrated how characterization of a symptom, in seven dimensions, provides information on the Where? (organ/system location) and the What? (pathological process) in the formula

Disease = Location + Pathological Process + Cause
         Where?   What?   Why?

This chapter carries the problem-solving process further by focusing on the third element in the formula—*Why? (cause).* As you interview, the detailed description of the symptoms begins to suggest *probabilities;* the weight of evidence is more consistent with disease in one system than another. Other symptoms suggest which pathological process may be present. The next step in the problem-centered interview gathers information from the patient's health history that suggests possible causal factors. We will also introduce for the first time a few concepts about how the interview, in addition to being a diagnostic tool, is an essential component in *treatment.*

☐ What is a Risk Factor?

A risk factor is any biological, psychosocial, or physical factor that predisposes to disease. Such factors include age and sex of the patient, prior illnesses that result in vulnerability to other disorders, hereditary and contagious mechanisms, and a wide spectrum of environmental hazards.

Risk factors have a statistical correlation with associated diseases of less than 1.0; they do not always result in disease. The correlation may be high, for example, the correlation between diabetes mellitus and arteriosclerotic vascular disease, or low as with the familial linkage of some forms of breast cancer. Many risk factors are synergistic, that is, several factors together cause disease; the exact contribution of each factor is rarely known (Goodman and Goodman, 1986). As more is learned about a disease mechanism, greater statistical correlation becomes possible.

For the clinician using the patient's history as a diagnostic tool, the most that can be practically achieved is identification of major risk factors in a patient's life, and some estimate of the probability that the risk factor is playing a role in the patient's condition. (In *Unit III: Health Promotion* we will consider how identifying risk factors helps prevent disease or leads to early diagnosis.)

Since statistics deal with groups of patients, the presence of a risk factor of 0.9 means that 9 out of 10 persons *at risk* will develop the condition—the patient you are interviewing may be the one person in 10 who does not become ill. You don't have to be an epidemiologist to make use of the risk factor concept. If your history-taking is thorough enough to identify the *presence* of significant risk factors, then the physical examination and specific laboratory testing can usually establish whether a possible risk factor is active. The challenge is not one of having the most precise statistical tables, it is simply discovering that risk factors are present.

The easiest way to demonstrate the practical use of the risk factor concept in clinical practice is to continue, from *Chapter 6: Symptoms Analysis*, the case of the 45-year-old man with retrosternal chest pain in whom symptom analysis of the Present Illness focused on the cardiovascular, respiratory, and gastrointestinal systems as the possible disease locations. Following symptom analysis, risk factors are identified by selectively exploring the patient's Past Health History, Family Health History, and Personal/Social History. As you continue the interview, several possibilities emerge.

If the patient has a Past Health History of chronic bronchitis with frequent occurrences of the same or similar type of symptoms, it suggests that the current problem may also be due to inflammation of the bronchi. A history of coronary artery disease (angina) or diabetes mellitus (which predisposes to coronary artery disease) would shift diagnostic interest to the cardiovascular system.

A patient whose Family Health History includes a number of relatives with respiratory disease suggests that your patient, too, has a similar condition. This could be a hereditary condition, or a contagious one such as tuberculosis.

A Personal/Social History of erratic eating habits, frequent and excessive alcohol consumption, and a liking for strong black coffee raises the possibility of esophageal or gastric irritation as the cause of the man's symptoms. Perhaps the patient has worked as a miner, an occupation with implications for chronic lung disease.

Here in more detail is a listing of the kinds of risk factors that enter into the diagnostic process and about which you inquire on a selective basis, as relevant.

☐ AGE, SEX, AND RACE

The implication of the risk factors of age, sex, and race is so pervasive that clinicians take them into account automatically. When writing up a clinical history or presenting a case to colleagues, clinicians invariably begin by stating the patient's age, sex, and race. These three facts immediately limit the range of diagnostic possibilities of many illnesses. Coronary artery disease, to cite one example, affects males far more often than females. Further, men begin to be affected in substantial numbers as early as age 35, whereas in women the condition is infrequent before menopause, which may not occur before age 45 to 50. Thus, if a 40-year-old patient with chest pain is a woman who has not reached the menopause, the chance of her pain being the result of coronary disease is less than if the patient were a man. On the other hand, if the patient with chest pain is a 20-year-old man, other conditions than coronary artery disease are likely. You will always deal with probabilities; however, 20-year-old men and 40-year-old women do get coronary artery disease. Problem-solving takes into account many factors other than probability.

The race of a patient is sometimes a risk factor. For example, when evaluating a patient with anemia, you would immediately consider sickle cell disease only if the patient is black. Black people also have a higher incidence of hypertension than do those of other races. The science of epidemiology studies populations of people to detect these differences, and then to search for the causative factors.

So great are the influences of age and sex, particularly, that two special-ties—pediatrics and obstetrics/gynecology—have areas of knowledge that are substantially separate from those of other specialties.

☐ OTHER RISKS

Past Health History. Relevant illnesses (chronic illness, past illness similar to present). Hospitalizations. Medications and immunizations. Menstrual his-tory.* General health before onset of the present illness.

Family Health History. Hereditary factors. Contagious elements.

Personal/Social History (Lifestyle). Social Relationships (spouse or partner, family, "significant others," friends, neighbors, support systems). Work

---

*Whether to classify menstrual history as a part of the Past Medical History or some other part of the history is arbitrary. Work out whatever scheme makes sense to you. The important thing is to include menstrual activity in *every interview* with a woman of childbearing age, regardless of the patient's problem.

(present & past), education. Recreation, hobbies, travel, sports. Personal habits (exercise, diet, caffeine consumption, alcohol consumption, sleep patterns, cigarette smoking, drug use and drug abuse). Sexual activity/ Preferences. Financial/Insurance. Spiritual, religious, philosophical beliefs.

Some risk factors, such as cigarette smoking or excessive alcohol consumption, are well known. You may wonder about some of the less obvious items on the list, such as recreation. Here are a few examples of recreation-related risk factors, and associated diseases:

Travel: Tropical diseases (malaria, amoebiasis, worms), deep-vein clots (thrombophlebitis) following prolonged sitting on airplanes.

Hobbies: Raising birds or animals (psitticosis, salmonella), cave exploration (fungal diseases), plastic arts (contact dermatitis).

Sports: Swimming (ear infections), musculoskeletal conditions like tendonitis or bursitis.

Music: Hearing loss in rock musicians.

Often, the patient fails to make the connection between some risk factor and the development of illness. A tropical illness, for example, may not develop for weeks after a patient has returned from a foreign land, and the patient may not think to mention the trip to you. Similarly, sports-related conditions may develop gradually and not be directly related to an acute injury during activity.

The Personal/Social History is a rich area for clues that may explain the patient's illness. The possibilities are enormous. Social relationships such as marital partner or friends, for example, have major implications for health and disease, yet many patients are reluctant to discuss social relationships unless given specific encouragement during the interview. Family violence, for example, is now recognized as a major public health problem involving the physical and mental health of victims, who may be children, adults, or the elderly (Check, 1985). Any type of social change may represent a significant loss for the patient.

A 54-year-old woman was admitted for an elective hysterectomy necessitated by uterine fibroids. She was visibly depressed. I noted on the chart that her birthdate had been the day before admission, and said, pleasantly enough I thought, "Happy birthday." The patient burst into tears. Several months ago her only son, of whom she was particularly fond, had married and moved to another town. He had always remembered his mother's birthday, but this time he did not. So the patient felt two "losses"—her uterus and her son.

A 55-year-old teacher had spent her entire professional life working with mentally retarded children. Over the years she had developed a special theory about teaching mentally retarded children, and somewhat unconsciously she had chosen a young boy as a test of her theory. One day the boy set fire to a wastebasket, and the teacher felt as if she had failed. "Thirty years of my life went up in smoke," she said. One week later she developed diabetes mellitus.

The link between life stresses and the onset of many types of illnesses has been recorded in a voluminous literature (Kaplan et al.), and the biological mechanisms are beginning to be understood (Weiner, 1984). Ader (1981), in a meticulous set of animal experiments, has demonstrated that the immune system can be influenced by simple conditioning experiments. Other links between mental phenomena and disease processes have been postulated to involve the hypothalamus-pituitary axis and the autonomic nervous system. The exact relationships are complex, and much research remains to be done, but the experience of many observant physicians convinces them that psychosocial factors play a significant role in disease (Eisenberg, 1980).

The workplace is the source of a wide variety of chronic illnesses. Some industrial illnesses, such as chronic lung disease related to asbestos exposure, may not develop for years after exposure. With American industry moving in the direction of high technology, new chemicals, radiation, and sophisticated industrial processes may be accompanied by new health hazards you will have to diagnose. Substance abuse, once confined to alcoholism, now involves drugs that appear in a variety of clinical disguises. Many of today's sexual practices are associated with serious health hazards, such as AIDS and other sexually transmitted diseases. Some alternate lifestyles are accompanied by bizarre diets and forms of natural healing that sooner or later bring patients to medical attention.

No physician discovers all the clues hidden in the patient's life history. Most difficulties do not arise from overlooking details, however, but from focusing entirely on the patient's symptoms and failing to consider risk factors at all. Only a few brief questions will survey major risk factors, and the benefits can be substantial, as reflected in this case.

A young woman, about 26, came to the emergency room one evening because of left upper quadrant pain. Her description was vague except for the location, and she had no other symptoms. She appeared to be well, but apprehensive. The vital signs recorded on the chart were all normal. The emergency service was busy that evening, and it was tempting to omit the Past, Family, and Personal/Social histories altogether, and do as brief an examination as possible. After all, the left upper quadrant is not a common site of significant symptoms, and she looked well.

Recalling that omitting major sections of the history had caused error in the past, the physician quickly surveyed the risk factors with just one openended question for each of the remaining sections. About Past Medical History, "Anything like this before?" "Yes, when I was 21, I had Hodgkin's disease, with an enlarged spleen that did cause me some pain where I have pain now. But they told me that treatment was successful, and all my check-ups since have been negative." Family Medical History was negative, but in asking who was in the family she mentioned that she had a two-month-old girl, her first child. Finally, regarding her Personal/Social *situation, she explained that her husband was in the Air Force and they had arrived at the base near town one month ago. One week ago her husband was unexpectedly transferred to special, and dangerous, duty.*

What initially appeared to be a minor symptom acquired a new meaning in the context of the patient with a history of Hodgkin's disease, a new mother, in a new city, and with her husband suddenly transferred to a dangerous situation. It is likely the patient was thinking, at some level of consciousness, "Now all I need is to have the Hodgkin's disease return."

Her examination was entirely normal; there was no evidence of spleen enlargement or abnormal nodes anywhere. I told her that my examination was negative. We talked briefly about what it was like to be in her situation. Just talking helped, and I'm sure she felt reassured by the fact that I had understood what was going on in her life. Had only her symptoms been evaluated, and risk factor assessment omitted, even the negative physical examination might not have addressed her concern.

□ Differential Diagnosis

Sometimes symptom analysis and risk factor identification leave no doubt about the disease causing the patient's illness. Often, however, you are left with several possibilities. The process of choosing from several diagnostic possibilities is termed *differential diagnosis:* a process of sorting out and weighing the evidence. Differential diagnosis is a form of the scientific method; initial data suggest several hypotheses, which are then confirmed or eliminated by additional data. Gradually one diagnostic hypothesis seems more likely than others. But even with a history strongly favoring one organ or system, you must gather added information from the physical examination and laboratory tests. If you are correct in your initial hypothesis, the added data strengthens or confirms your impression. Sometimes, however, even after a complete evaluation, you are still uncertain about the diagnosis, and may have to treat the patient based only on a probable diagnosis.

□ Risk Factors and Probability

Useful as is the identification of risk factors in problem solving, it has a lower priority than carefully analyzing the *Present Illness*. The reason has to do with probability. Knowing that a risk factor is present does not necessarily mean it is active. In each of the above examples there exists only a possibility that the common sense connection is the correct explanation. Sometimes a common sense explanation turns out to be wrong, or only partially correct—to paraphrase

H.L. Mencken, "There is no human problem, however complex, for which an explanation cannot be found that is simple, clear, direct—and wrong."

Another problem with risk factors in diagnosis is that the cause of most diseases is an incompletely understood chain of events. Coronary artery disease, for example, reflects genetic, dietary, metabolic, and psychological mechanisms, tobacco use, age- and sex-related elements, and other interacting factors. Medical science has not reached a stage of sophistication in which all factors are known, or the contribution of each to the pathological process of myocardial infarction understood.

Given the current state of medical knowledge, the best that is possible with regard to causation is establishing probabilities. A male over age 40 with diabetes mellitus, in whose family there is a high prevalence of coronary artery disease, who smokes, eats fatty foods, and is driven by ambition, time-pressure, and competition (the "type A" personality) is more likely to suffer a myocardial infarction than a man without any of these characteristics. Exactly when the infarction will happen, if it happens at all, cannot be predicted. And even if it does happen, the exact contribution of each of the factors is not known. (Not all diagnoses are so problematic. If you happen to get in the way of a speeding car, it does not require exceptional diagnostic skill to determine the probable cause of the sudden development of multiple fractures.)

□ Errors of Logic

If you've ever had a course in logic you will easily recognize how logical errors can mislead your diagnostic thinking (Fulginiti, 1981). One fallacy—*post hoc, ergo propter hoc,* "after, therefore because of"—is at work whenever a risk factor so dominates the clinical picture that "common sense" leads you to believe it is the cause of a condition. A Past Medical History of bronchitis, for example, in no way keeps a patient from developing a new condition, such as coronary artery disease. Nor does a Family Medical History of respiratory disease mean that your patient could not develop a heart condition. And not everyone who eats irregularly and drinks large amounts of alcohol or coffee develops gastrointestinal disease.

Examples such as these suggest that you should not let the presence of risk factors and the search for causes exercise too great an influence over your diagnostic thinking. The most useful data come from carefully considering *manifestations* of disease—the Present Illness expressed as symptoms and signs. Often this information is sufficient to allow you to arrive at a reasonable formulation about the nature of the underlying disease without relying upon the somewhat uncertain implications of risk factors.

The following example, from another field altogether—investigation of aircraft accidents—illustrates how easy it is to jump to a wrong conclusion.

A commercial airliner crashed at a time of intense thunderstorm activity.

The pilot was on probationary status because of several incidents in which he had exercised poor judgment, including flying in unsafe weather. The airline had one of the worst safety records in the industry, and was near bankruptcy.

Several risk factors seem to be possible causes of the crash: a violent storm, an incompetent pilot, poor airline management. The first step in any aircraft accident investigation, however, is reconstructing the airplane from the wreckage. When this was done, it was clear that the airplane had been blown apart by an explosive; traces of dynamite were on the inside of numerous metal fragments from the baggage compartment of the plane. The investigation then turned up the fact one passenger carried a large amount of air accident insurance, taken out by her husband, who was not on the plane. He confessed to placing dynamite with a timing device in her luggage. Despite several "obvious" causes for the crash, the truth could only have been learned by the analysis of the wreckage of the airplane—the Present Illness.

Here are two clinical situations in which a risk factor could have so dominated the clinical picture that the true diagnosis might not have become immediately evident.

Shoveling snow imposes heavy physical and thermal demands on the cardiovascular system, and myocardial infarction (heart attack) is common in the snowbelt. The morning after the first heavy snowfall I received an urgent call from a man who six months previously had had an infarction. Recently, he had felt so well that he decided to clear his driveway of snow the previous night.

He awoke the next morning with chest pain. Both of us were understandably concerned. Before sending for an ambulance, however, I asked him to describe his pain over the phone. I then relaxed. His pain was over the breast areas, aggravated by arm movement and nothing else. He had no cardiovascular symptoms. I asked him to press firmly over the pectorales muscles. Yes, they were tender. The answer, of course, was nothing more serious than muscle soreness from unaccustomed exercise. A hurried question or two about chest pain, instead of a careful Sacred Seven evaluation, might have resulted in an unnecessary and expensive heart evaluation. In most instances, even semi-emergencies, a clear description of the current symptoms is the best insurance against diagnostic error. In this case the risk factor of myocardial infarction (Past Medical History) was not a causal element in this episode of illness.

A 45-year-old woman, well known to her physicians for her frequent alcoholic excesses, developed jaundice. Cirrhosis of the liver was the obvious explanation, but an impacted gallstone was the actual cause. The jaundice turned out to be due to obstruction of the bile duct resulting from a small impacted gallstone.

A careful history will help you avoid incorrect conclusions. The snow shoveler's chest pains, when carefully described, were altogether unlike those associated with heart disease, but quite consistent with simple muscle pain; the woman with the history of alcoholism gave a clear description of gallbladder colic the day before the onset of the jaundice. It is safer to first analyze the patient's problem in terms of structure and pathological process before looking for risk elements that suggest an initiating cause. This principle was expressed by a great neurologist, Hughlings Jackson, who said, "The search for the cause of a thing should await a description of the thing being caused."

□ Risk Factors and Treatment

Thus far, the focus has been on the diagnostic value of risk factors. No interview is entirely diagnostic, however. As you search for diagnostic elements, you also come across information that influences treatment once the diagnosis is established.

Past Medical History. Existing illness, such as diabetes, heart disease, or depression, will influence treatment of a new condition. Current medications and medication allergies may create an adverse reaction if new drugs are prescribed.

Family Medical History. Contagious illness, or the presence of a family member who is at risk because of immunosuppression or chronic illness, which could be aggravated by the patient's illness, may make the situation more serious.

Personal/Social History (Lifestyle). What social supports (family, friends, community organizations, church) does the patient have? The ability to work depends on the effect of continuing to work on the patient and on the nature of the work (nursing, responsibility for others). Recreation is a form of mental and physical therapy. Personal habits (diet, alcohol, coffee, tobacco (smoking when recovering from bronchitis) may affect the condition. Sexual activity may be a concern (after a heart attack, for example). What is the patient's financial status (ability to afford continuing health care after a major illness which results in job loss)? This information should also be included in a *health promotion* interview. What are the patient's spiritual beliefs (support, Last Rites, dietary restrictions)?

A few examples will highlight how risk factors have implications for treatment.

A painter in his 30's falls from a ladder, lands on his head, and is unconscious for two or three minutes. A careful examination by the emergency room physician reveals no evidence of brain injury. The most likely diagnosis is concussion, but intracranial bleeding can never be ruled out. The next step is close observation by a family member—awakening the patient every two hours to determine level of consciousness. The painter, however, lives alone and has no friends who could stay with him overnight. Therefore, the patient is admitted to the hospital for observation.

A young woman with a long history of cystic acne consults her physician because the condition is worsening and she wants to cure it if possible. Here there is no question about the diagnosis. However, in quickly checking her Past Medical History, the physician learns that she has missed two menstrual periods and may be pregnant. An effective treatment for pustular acne is isotretinoin, but the drug is teratogenic (capable of producing deformities of the embryo) and contraindicated in pregnancy.

Work hazards are a significant risk factor in some illnesses, such as low back pain in a heavy-construction worker. Conversely, the illness must also be considered in the context of the patient's work; for example, a nurse with a communicable respiratory disease should be advised not to return to work until over the illness.

The financial status of your patients is a risk factor you will need to consider. Patients with little or no insurance are at great risk should serious illness occur: they may not be able to afford necessary care. It is not unusual for patients to fail to fill a prescription because they didn't have the money to buy it. Many people are too proud to admit their financial difficulties.

Another facet of lifestyle rarely thought about—spiritual, religious, and philosophical beliefs—is at times relevant to the care of patients. Refusal of some religious groups to provide basic immunizations for their children or to permit administration of blood or blood products will have significant impact on the care you provide. Christian Science minimizes the role of conventional medical care, and many alternative lifestyles prevalent these days may go to dangerous extremes of diet, natural cures, and exclusive reliance on mental attempts to control illness.

Various religions frequently have specific rituals or observances with health care significance. Last Rites are an essential part of the Catholic religion; should a Catholic patient die without a priest having been called, the family will find it hard to forgive you. Even religious dietary observances have, on occasion, implications for the health care you provide.

A woman in her 60's was admitted because of a hip fracture requiring surgery. The surgery and postoperative course were uneventful, but the patient started to lose substantial weight. The problem: she was an orthodox Jew who observed Kosher dietary laws that defined the kinds of foods permitted, and even the kinds of plates on which food could be served. The hospital kitchen was not Kosher, of course. She was too reticent to make her needs known—she just stopped eating.

☐ Practical Questions: Getting Risk Factor Data

All this may be more than you bargained for. You cannot consider the entire life history of every patient you see before making diagnostic and therapeutic decisions. Fortunately, this is not always necessary. Many illnesses are what they appear to be, and their diagnosis and treatment are straightforward. But there are patients for whom your knowledge of risk factors will make an important difference in their diagnosis and treatment.

You need to have a reliable, systematic procedure that alerts you to these patients. If you are in a practice in which continuity of care provides opportunities to get to know your patients, you'll have the background information without having to ask each time you see the patient. For patients who are new to you, the primary safeguard is simply the *Fundamental Four*; a habitual consideration, however brief, of Past Medical History, Family Medical History, and Personal/Social History in addition to the Present Illness. A quick overview takes a very few minutes (much less time than is consumed by care based on an incorrect diagnosis resulting from lack of essential information), *provided* you consider these areas at all. You'll intuitively know what topics need to be explored in detail. In addition, simple checklists, questionnaires completed by the patient, and computers all have a place in data gathering and are discussed in *Unit VIII: Technical Supports.*

☐ REFERENCES AND READINGS

Ader R: Psychoneuroimmunology. New York, Academic Press, 1981.

Check WA: Homicide, suicide, other violence gain increasing medical attention. 'Public health problem' of violence receives epidemiological attention. JAMA (Medical News) 1985;254:721–730, 881–892.

Cohen MF: Domestic violence. Med Law 1985;4:19–27.

Eisenberg L: What makes persons "patients" and patients "well?" Am J Med 1980;69:277–285.

Fulginiti VA: Pediatric Clinical Problem Solving. Baltimore, Williams & Wilkins, 1981, pp 47–54.

Goodman LE, Goodman MJ: Prevention—how misuse of a concept undercuts its worth. Hastings Center Report 1986; April:26–38.

Kaplan HI et al: Psychological factors affecting physical conditions (psychosomatic disorders). In Kaplan HI, Sadock BJ (eds): Comprehensive Textbook of Medicine IV, ed 4. Baltimore, Williams & Wilkins, 1985, pp 1106–1219.

Lasswell AB, Roe DA, Hochheiser L: Nutritional assessment and assessment tools. In: Nutrition for Family and Primary Care Practitioners. Philadelphia, George F Stickley Company, 1986, chap 3.

Levy BS, Wegman DH: The occupational history in medical practice. Postgrad Med 1986;79:301–311.

Millman RB: Drug abuse and drug dependence. In Frances AJ, Hales RE (eds): Annual Review, Vol 5. Washington DC, American Psychiatric Press, 1986, pp 120–227.

Occupational Health Committee: Taking the occupational history. Ann Intern Med 1983;99:641–651.

Weiner H: The prospects for psychosomatic medicine. Psychosomatic Med 1984;44:491–517.

Wulf HR: Rational Diagnosis and Treatment, 2nd ed. London, Blackwell Scientific Publications, 1981.

CHAPTER 9

THE PROBLEM-CENTERED INTERVIEW

Mini-Database

Having discussed symptom analysis and risk factors, let's assemble the parts. The *Problem-Centered* history consists of a detailed description of the patient's symptoms plus *relevant* facts from the Past Health History, Family Health History, and Personal/Social History. This is the heart of the interview, and of the diagnostic process. Obtaining the Problem-Centered history is difficult and challenging because of uncertainty about what is relevant. With experience, your sense of relevance will strengthen.

☐ The *Fundamental Four*

The patient's history consists of four major classes of information, *The Fundamental Four*:
1. Present Illness.*
2. Past Health History.
3. Family Health History (Hereditary/Contagious History). ⎫ Risk Factors
4. Personal/Social History. ⎭

You'll meet the *Fundamental Four* again. Both a Problem-Centered and a Health Promotion interview follow the same outline. The first is short and selective; the second long and detailed. The distinction between the two basic

---

*Great variability exists in the terms used to describe this aspect of the patient's history. Other terms include *Chief Complaint* and *History of the Present Illness*.

interview types is discussed in *Unit III: Health Promotion.* A traditional fifth category, the *Review of Systems,* is logically a part of the Present Illness and is discussed in *Chapter 7: Review of Systems.*

Here is a detailed, step-by-step outline of the problem-centered history.

□ What to Learn from the Patient

□ BROAD PICTURE

First get an introductory, unstructured overview, from the patient's point of view, of the current problem, its setting, how it evolves over time, and importance to patient. Answers to your *open-ended* request, "Tell me more about it," help you decide on the subsequent course of the interview. It is insurance against false starts or missing the patient's main concern. Ask the patient to "begin at the beginning." Another good lead-in question is, "When were you last *entirely* well?" This may detect the beginning of subtle, but ignored, symptoms which only later caused enough concern that the patient decided to consult a doctor. For example, a patient, first seen because of a myocardial infarction (heart attack), may have had chest pain (due to gradually narrowing coronary arteries) for months or years. The beginning of the *Present Illness* thus is long before the heart attack.

Present Illness

Ask what is currently wrong. Get a clear description of the major symptom or cluster of symptoms. A broad overview of the patient's present illness is followed by symptom analysis in these dimensions:
1. Location.
2. Quality.
3. Timing/Chronology.
4. Severity.
5. Setting/Onset.
6. Modifying factors ("Better/Worse").
7. Associated symptoms (Relevant Review of Systems).

□ Causal or Risk Factors

Past Health History. Find out about *relevant* illnesses (chronic illness, past illness similar to present), prolonged care, hospitalizations, immunizations, medication history and, for females, menstrual history.* Also ask about the patient's general health before onset of the present illness.

Family Health History. Are there hereditary diseases in the family? Determine the contagious health history.

Personal/Social History (Lifestyle). Find out about social relationships (i.e., family, significant others, friends, neighbors, and support systems), work (present/past), education, recreation/hobbies/travel, personal habits (i.e., exercise, dietary habits, sleep patterns, caffeine and alcohol consumption, cigarette smoking, recreational drug use), sexual activity/preferences, financial/insurance resources, spiritual/religious/philosophical beliefs.

Three Final Questions

1. Anything else to add?
2. Your ideas and concerns about the current problem?
3. Anything you'd like to ask about?

When you boil it all down, these are the questions (whether the answers come from the patient, chart, or others who know the patient) that enable you to determine:

□ *What is going on right now?* (Present Illness)
□ *Has anything like this happened before?* (Past Medical History)
□ *Has anything like this happened in the family or to close friends?* (Family Medical History)
□ *Is lifestyle influencing health?* (Personal/Social History)

□ A MAN WITH BACKACHE: A MINI-DATABASE

Consider, for example, a 24-year-old man with a complaint of "back pain." The Problem-Centered history looks like this:

Present Illness

Current Problem: Back pain
1. **Location:** Mid-lumbar area occasionally radiating to the right thigh and leg.

---

*The menstrual history can be a part of the Present Illness or the Past Medical History. The decision about classification is arbitrary. What is important is asking every woman of childbearing age about this dimension of health and illness. From the diagnostic standpoint, early pregnancy simulates other diseases or may worsen pre-existing conditions such as diabetes. Diagnostic procedures such as x-rays are potentially harmful, as are the effects of therapies, especially medications, on the early fetus.

2. **Quality:** Dull "pulling" sensation.

3. **Timing/Chronology:** Duration 3 days, worse by evening, better in the a.m.

4. **Severity:** "Moderate," but couldn't go to work today because of the discomfort.

5. **Setting/Onset:** Gradual onset the day after working in a large garden.

6. **Modifying Factors:** Worse with movement, getting into a car, coughing. Better when lying quietly on his back. Tylenol helps.

7. **Associated Symptoms:** Musculoskeletal ROS: Stiffness, local back tenderness.

   Peripheral Nervous System (ROS): No weakness/sensory change.[1]
   Systemic ROS: No fever.[2]

Relevant Past Health History

Good general health. No prior back pain, no arthritis.[3] Drug allergy: Aspirin causes a rash.

Relevant Family Health History

Mother has a long history of back trouble. Brother has had back surgery.

Relevant Personal/Social History

☐ Social history: The patient lives alone.
☐ Work: A salesman during the week, manages a small farm on weekends.
☐ Recreation: Bowling.
☐ Financial: No health insurance.

☐ Pertinent Negatives

In this example there are three "pertinent negatives," facts that *tend to eliminate* one of the diagnostic possibilities:

1. Suggests no involvement of the peripheral nervous system.
2. Tends to rule out infection as a pathological process.
3. Suggests this is not a chronic or recurrent problem.

If the patient's initial description suggests the possibility of urinary system involvement, the absence of burning or frequent urination, or of bloody or cloudy urine tends to eliminate the urinary system as the source of back pain.

In every problem-solving situation think about *relevant* data from the Review of Systems, Past Health History, Family Health History, and Personal/Social History which, if present, favors a specific diagnosis and if absent tend to eliminate a diagnostic possibility. This approach to problem solving, known as differential diagnosis, is discussed in *Chapter 8: Risk Factors in Diagnosis and Treatment.*

□ Relevance: How Much Data to Collect in a Problem-Centered Interview?

In this history of a patient having back pain, many areas of health history were *not* asked about: childhood illness, vision, hearing, presence of heart disease in the family, personal habits such as smoking or alcohol, and many other topics that would be a part of a comprehensive history. While such information would be significant in the context of other medical problems, or Health Promotion, they are not relevant to the problem of back pain.

You are never certain about what is relevant and what can be omitted in a Problem-Centered interview, however. Since the kidneys are a frequent source of back pain, it would be reasonable to include the urinary system in the relevant *Review of Systems* (Associated Symptoms); negative responses would be "pertinent negatives." Because of the uncertainty about relevance, you should complement the Problem-Centered history with a Health Promotion history as soon as possible. Sometimes you will learn information relevant to the patient's problem while doing the Health Promotion interview—for example, the patient may recall under the heading of Past Health History a childhood illness that the doctor thought "might be polio, which could cause back trouble later on." Several different ways to complete the history are discussed in *Chapter 13: A Combined Problem-Centered/Health Promotion Interview.*

If some area of the history does not seem relevant, yet you are uneasy about omitting it altogether, start with a broad, open-ended question. For example, you may feel the urinary system is an unlikely source of the back pain, yet a possibility. The most general question you could ask is "How are your kidneys and bladder?" or "Are you having problems with urination?" A positive response would signal the need for further questioning in this area; a negative response terminates this area of inquiry.

Questions dealing with areas of lifestyle, such as personal relationships, sexual behavior, finances, and habits may seem to the patient to be inappropriate or intrusive unless you point out the relevance of what you are asking. If you sense an area may be a sensitive one, preface your question with a brief explanation:

"Sometimes, Mr. Jones, stress in a marriage can lead to the kind of problem you are having. How is your marriage situation?"

□ Getting More Information

As you review the information you acquire from the patient during the initial interview, new diagnostic possibilities often come to mind. You find you need to explore areas that you skipped the first time. This is a normal event in any kind of problem-solving task. If you look at the situation from the standpoint of the scientific method, you will recognize that a problem-solving interview involves hypothesis formation, testing, selectively acquiring more information, reformulating the hypothesis, and more information collection until you have solved the problem. When evaluating patients, you have data from the history, physical examination, laboratory tests, and response to initial therapy (see Therapeutic Trial, *Chapter 10: Diagnostic Strategies*) upon which to develop your diagnostic hypothesis. Unlike a scientific experiment, you cannot obtain more information anytime you recognize the need. You have to await another opportunity to be with the patient. If the patient is in the hospital, returning for more information is a simple matter. If the patient was seen in a medical office, you may have to wait for the patient's next visit. Sometimes you can get the needed information in the patient's record, or by calling the patient. In any event, do not feel that you should have obtained all the information the first time. The diagnostic process is frequently a complex challenge, and no one, however experienced, can anticipate the precise information requirements of problem solving.

□ MICROANALYSIS

A productive technique of getting additional information is to ask the patient to go back over sections of the history and add details that might have been omitted the first time. Like solving a detective mystery, the clues may need a more precise account of the illness. Any part of the history may contain the information needed to reach a correct diagnosis when the initial history fails to explain the patient's condition. Robinson (1984) tells of a 50-year-old man, a motel manager, who some years before had been diagnosed by another physician as having angina (chest pains associated with coronary artery disease) and given nitroglycerin to take whenever he had chest pain. Although an electrocardiogram showed only non-specific abnormalities, the history the patient gave was typical of angina: "Why, I can't even make it across my motel parking lot without stopping to take a nitroglycerin tablet." One day while aboard an airliner, he developed severe chest pain, and discovered that he had forgotten to take his nitroglycerin along. The cabin attendant, having nothing better to offer, tried an antacid, with miraculous and immediate relief. Thereafter, the patient abandoned the nitroglycerin, since he invariably obtained full relief with the antacid. Robinson continues

Still bewildered by the entire situation, I felt compelled to resort to a basic technique: history taking. "Tell me more about walking across the motel parking lot. What does that involve?" "Well," he said, "I frequently walk across the parking lot to check the rooms ... I usually bend over to pick up the trash as I go. Come to think of it, that is when I get the chest pain."

An exercise tolerance test of the heart was completely normal, with no evidence of coronary artery disease. But an X-ray of the upper gastrointestinal tract (upper GI series) showed a large hernia of the diaphragm with esophageal spasm, diagnostic of esophageal reflux, a condition that often mimics angina and is frequently brought on by bending or other movements that increase intra-abdominal pressure. The key to the correct diagnosis was in a micro-detailed description of exactly what was going on at the onset of symptoms.

□ Time Pressure: The *Fundamental Four*—The Safe Minimum

The Problem-Centered mini-database described in this chapter can be accomplished in a short time. Yet, when under pressure, the temptation is strong to omit the risk factors and just concentrate on the Present Illness (current symptoms). The time saved is not worth the possibility of omitting important, sometimes crucial information.

A 10-month-old infant was seen because of moderate diarrhea lasting three days. Simple home remedies were of no help. The mother noticed that the child was urinating only small amounts of urine and was becoming seriously dehydrated.

The case seemed simple enough. The symptoms all pointed to a diagnosis of diarrhea with dehydration. The child was examined, found to be dehydrated, and was hospitalized. The infant responded to care, and was discharged in 48 hours.

Had the interviewer taken another minute to go through the Fundamental Four, *and had asked a single question covering* Family Medical History *("Anything like this in your family or friends?"), the fact of a small epidemic would have emerged. Two older brothers also had diarrhea, but were not ill enough to need medical help. Further, the next door neighbor's family was also experiencing diarrhea. As it turned out, a contaminated neighborhood water supply was causing the bacterial diarrhea.*

Always touch base with each of the major sections of the *Fundamental Four*. Often you'll learn all you need to know with just a single, open-ended question for each section mentioned at the beginning of the chapter:

☐ Anything like this before? (Past Medical History)
☐ Anything like this in the family or among close friends? (Family Medical History)
☐ Is Lifestyle influencing health? (Personal/Social History)

The problem-solving process is a *selective* evaluation, and requires constant decisions about what to ask and what to omit. This selective approach is the most difficult, challenging, and exciting aspect of interviewing. Problem-solving of this sort is the essence of the diagnostic process and the activity that occupies the greatest amount of the clinician's time with patients.

☐ Treatment

Imbedded in diagnostic information is data that is relevant to treatment. The 24-year-old man with backache is allergic to aspirin, therefore aspirin-containing medications, which might be adequate for pain control, have to be avoided. Since he lived alone, he might not be able to manage the prescribed bed rest unless he was in the hospital, but he had no hospital insurance. For the child with diarrhea, management affected the entire neighborhood. The Health Department was notified, and the contaminated water line was quickly shut off.

In theory, clinical problem-solving would seem to be separate from treatment. In practice, the two cannot be entirely separated. Blois (1985) comments:

We do act as though there were separate compartments labeled "diagnosis" and "treatment," and later "follow-up." This is almost certainly not the case; there is probably no time when a physician thinks of diagnosis and nothing else—nor is there any later period when diagnosis is not thought of at all. A diagnosis can always be modified or changed, depending on the patient's response to treatment.

☐ The Complex Problem Environment

Patients frequently have multiple problems. At times you will feel like a juggler as you keep an eye on each while maintaining an effective overall patient care plan. As you acquire experience you'll find yourself comfortably handling several problems at the same times. Much depends on your ability to keep efficient charts detailing what is happening to your patients. This subject is discussed in *Chapter 27: Records and Written Communications*. Multiple diagnoses is discussed in *Chapter 10: Diagnostic Strategies*.

Sometimes as one problem is resolved another problem emerges:

A commercial airplane crashed on take-off. There were survivors. One man, it turned out, had a crash-related problem that became progressively more serious the better his injuries healed. He lived in a distant city, and as he left on a business trip he had made a point of telling his wife that he would be somewhere other than his true destination. He was having an affair. The first his wife knew about his true whereabouts was when she received a call from the hospital.

In the early days of his hospitalization, his burns and fractures were the major focus, but as these improved, it became apparent that he faced a break-up of his marriage. The two problems could not be separated.

□ Prevention

In the next unit, *Health Promotion,* prevention and early detection of disease will be discussed. The distinction between problem-centered and health promotion interviews is not a clear one, since an important element of any treatment plan is to anticipate and, if possible, prevent complications. Here are a few examples of how prevention is an essential part of treatment.

Patients with diabetes mellitus are subject to a variety of complications, including severe retinal disease (diabetes mellitus is the leading cause of acquired blindness in this country). When diabetes mellitus is diagnosed, good medical management includes a referral to an ophthalmologist, even if the patient has no current vision complaints, for initial evaluation and periodic re-examination. If early evidence of diabetic inflammation of the retina is discovered, laser photocoagulation can minimize visual impairment and preserve sight.

Pneumococci bacteria cause serious pneumonia and life-threatening meningitis. Persons at risk for these conditions include children who have had surgical removal of the spleen and older persons with chronic respiratory diseases. A readily available vaccine (polyvalent pneumococcal vaccine) provides substantial protection against pneumococcal infections and should be a part of the treatment of persons at risk.

□ Conclusion

The Sacred Seven and the *Fundamental Four* are the essence of the problem-centered interview. If you understand these two concepts, you'll never get lost during an interview. With the *Fundamental Four* you gradually build a balanced clinical history that serves the purpose of problem-solving. Without such a framework to guide you, it is easy to be overwhelmed with details of uncertain significance. You work harder but have less to show for it. Seeing the overall picture, on the other hand, allows you to decide which details are worth getting. In interviewing, as in many other things, the comment of Ludwig Mies van der Rohe, an architect who pioneered simplicity in building design, is worth considering:

"Less is more."

□ REFERENCES

Blois M: The physician's personal workstation. M.D. Computing 1985;2:22–26.
Robinson NJ: The history that wasn't. NC Med J 1984;45:650.

CHAPTER 10

NON-ANALYTIC DIAGNOSTIC STRATEGIES

The problem-solving method described in the previous chapters of this unit—Think Organs/Systems and determine *location, pathological process,* and *cause*—is a rational, analytic approach to diagnosis, but is not the only diagnostic method. Clinicians use a variety of problem-solving strategies, some of which are described in this chapter.

☐ Early Diagnosis

One reason for the importance of non-analytic diagnostic methods is that people often are seen early in the course of their illness, sometimes within hours of its onset when only non-specific clinical manifestations are present. Before health care services were readily available (and in many parts of the world even today), people used to wait days or weeks before seeking health care. By then the diagnosis was usually clear because of the advanced stage of the disease. For example, the early manifestations of meningitis often are no different than those of many other infections—fever, chills, fatigue, and headache. The stiff neck, mental confusion, shock, and other signs of meningitis may not develop until later, and unfortunately when cure is difficult and sometimes impossible.

☐ Pattern Recognition

Experienced clinicians often arrive at a correct diagnosis "at a glance." This ability, called *intuition, hunch,* or *pattern recognition,* involves an unconscious but powerful ability to observe and integrate a spectrum of clinical clues, and it becomes increasingly accurate as your experience with patients accumulates. Even your failures improve this skill. Each new patient, correctly diagnosed or not, adds to your inventory of experiences against which to compare new ones.

Sometimes you may not know exactly what is wrong with a patient, but have a feeling that something about the patient is different or unfamiliar. Respect such intuitions—often they tell you something important.

A 52-year-old woman was seen on a busy day in February. The day was busy because an epidemic of "flu" was in full force. Patient after patient had the same symptoms: aching muscles and mild fever. Initially, this patient was no different—she ached and had a fever. After a few minutes, however, she somehow seemed unlike the other "flu" patients. As it turned out, she had dermatomyositis, a relatively rare collagen-vascular disease. What was different about her was this: as we finished the interview and she got up to go to the examination room, she gave a slight push on the arms of the chair. She was developing proximal muscle weakness, characteristic of dermatomyositis but not of "flu." Although she had not mentioned weakness as a symptom, the uniqueness of her nonverbal actions somehow signaled that she didn't fit the usual picture of a "flu" patient.

We unconsciously process subtle differences all the time. Think of your ability to recognize at a glance a friend you haven't seen in years. Radiologists look at an X-ray film for a few seconds and spot an abnormality that may be difficult for you to appreciate even when it is pointed out. The radiologist does not deliberately examine every shadow on the X-ray, but processes the entire image at an unconscious level and somehow recognizes the abnormal area to be more closely examined. Here is another example of the power of pattern recognition:

A 42-year-old man had been seen in April for initial evaluation of hypertension. He returned a month later for a complete examination. As he started to remove his necktie, he paused, and then said, "Oh, by the way, ever since I was here last, I've had a rash," and he made a sweeping gesture that indicated the rash was all over his chest. "Would you mind taking a look at it?" Pityriasis rosea, a very mild skin condition, immediately flashed into mind and proved to be the correct diagnosis. How was a rash diagnosed before seeing it or taking any kind of history? The major clue was probably his casual, "Oh, by the way. . . ." Also, his apologetic manner suggested that the rash wasn't causing significant symptoms or concern. The four-week duration and the springtime occurrence, also characteristic of pityriasis rosea, added to the unconscious mental processing that lead to the correct diagnosis.

□ The Textbook Case—A Rarity

Any one patient rarely fits a "textbook" or "classic" disease pattern. Such patients often attract a lot of attention—doctors and students are invited to see the patient—because they are rare. Patients vary enormously in how they manifest a disease, especially in the early stages. Forcing the patient's illness to fit a preconceived pattern frequently results in a missed diagnosis. It is much safer to analyze the patient's problem in stages, first determining the organ or system involved, then defining the pathological process and searching for causal factors.

A woman in her twenties had experienced gradually worsening muscular weakness over a four year period. First her legs became weak and later the weakness spread to her arms. She was examined by many neurologists and internists, none of whom could explain her condition. As is often the case when no medical diagnosis is established, a psychological condition such as hysteria is diagnosed by exclusion. Fortunately, the woman was finally evaluated by a neurologist who had extensive experience with myasthenia gravis (a rare but well-known muscle disorder described in every textbook of medicine). He immediately suspected an atypical manifestation of this disease, and his diagnosis was confirmed when an injection of an anticholinesterase medication resulted in almost immediate, although temporary, return of full strength.

One of the first physicians to examine the patient had considered myasthenia gravis in the differential diagnosis, but failed to follow up this lead because he remembered reading that the symptoms of myasthenia gravis develop first in the head and face muscles, not in the legs. The neurologist who made the correct diagnosis commented, "It is sad to think how close she came to an early diagnosis . . . (One physician) suspected myasthenia gravis, but he made the mistake of going entirely by the book. The books all emphasize that the presenting symptoms are drooping eyelids, facial weakness, palatal weakness and difficulty speaking. Classical teaching requires the presence of one or more of those symptoms for a diagnosis of myasthenia . . . I wish the textbooks were a little less rigid. But the fact is that a mere suspicion of myasthenia is enough, because there's a quick and easy diagnostic test that is almost entirely reliable."

(Roueche, 1984)

□ Zebras

Thinking first of exceedingly rare conditions is a special hazard of university medical centers. Perri Klass (1985), while a third year medical student, describes the trap this way:

The idea is that when a normal person (not a medical student or doctor) hears hoofbeats, the first thought that comes to mind is "horse." But a medical student hears hoofbeats and immediately thinks "zebra!" Medical students, the cliche goes, think first about the rare, unlikely diagnosis and are uninterested in common medical problems. The medical student not only expects those hoofbeats to be a zebra, but is actually disappointed to see no exotic black and white stripes, just a plain old horse. And the fact is, the appeal of the rare and dramatic disease is built right into medical training. . . .

Teaching hospitals are places to which community physicians refer patients with rare and unfamiliar conditions. Often one member of the faculty is an authority in some infrequent condition. Thus, the patient population of a university hospital is unlikely to reflect the typical prevalence of illnesses in the community. Difficulties arise only if you let the case mix in a university setting, where you receive your first clinical experience, bias your diagnostic judgment when you work in a community setting. The best cure for the zebra syndrome is a clerkship in a community hospital, or spending some time with a primary care physician. These experiences put rare and unusual conditions in perspective and result in a more balanced medical education.

☐ Semantic Diagnosis

As you become more experienced in diagnosis, you will find yourself moving away from the *Think Systems* approach to a disease-oriented diagnostic process based on symptoms, physical findings, and laboratory results. This method involves the matching of the patient's illness with the characteristics of a textbook description of disease. Physicial findings often add a degree of specificity, and some laboratory tests are more specific still.

Often the process deteriorates into what could be called semantic diagnosis: a superficial form of diagnosis, or pseudodiagnosis, based entirely on words. This approach involves *matching* sets of words that describe a patient's illness with words physicians use to identify diseases. Words and phrases become equated with the disease. Sometimes a single phrase is all that is cited, for example:

morning sickness = early pregnancy

poor eye contact = schizophrenia

butterfly rash = lupus erythematosus

Sometimes sets of medical terms are joined together to identify diseases:

polydipsia, polyphagia, polyuria = diabetes mellitus

early morning awakening, constipation, loss of
appetite and libido = depression

Just as patients fail to fit textbook descriptions of disease, neither do they fit brief semantic formulas. Also, subtle nonverbal information often escapes conscious detection and is not included in discussions. The risk is greatest in medical centers where teaching involves much more discussion than in-depth, continuing patient contact. (Time-study evaluation of teaching rounds shows that lecturing and rounds may take up more than 90 per cent of the time spent in clinical teaching.) The more time you spend with patients, the less you will be swayed by semantic diagnosis.

We all need to use words to communicate, of course, and a part of the diagnostic process is correlating the patient's clinical manifestations with descriptions of typical diseases. But words are easy to misuse. If you remain aware of when words identify biological phenomena and when they simply refer to other words, your diagnostic skills will remain fresh and accurate.

□ Syndromes

The term *syndrome* refers to a set of symptoms, physical findings, and laboratory findings that uniquely characterize a single disease. This definition overlaps with the definition of *disease,* but does have several unique meanings. One refers to genetic disorders that uniformly display specific clinical manifestations, often involving multiple systems. For example, Marfan's syndrome includes abnormalities of the eyes, arms and legs, the aorta, and other organs; some people believe Abraham Lincoln had Marfan's syndrome. Another way in which syndrome is used is to designate a seemingly new and not yet well understood disease. *Toxic shock* and *AIDS* had both been called syndromes, but as their pathophysiological mechanisms became understood they have been designated diseases. If syndromes were illnesses with uniform manifestations and were fully developed from their onset, the term might serve a useful diagnostic and therapeutic purpose. Most syndromes, however, are defined only after someone recognizes a unique pattern in many patients, each of whom initially experienced only some of the syndrome's manifestations; thus, the concept is not often useful in early diagnosis. (Until recently, a syndrome was likely to be named after the scientist who first recognized the pattern; medical dictionaries are filled with hundreds of syndromes named after their discoverers.)

□ One Disease or Several?

The diagnostic process gets really complex when a patient has several co-existing diseases. In clinical diagnosis, as in the scientific method generally, the diagnostician strives to explain all the disease manifestations with a single diagnosis. In the scientific method this is the *Law of Parsimony*. The fact is, however, that many patients have multiple diseases, each contributing to the set of symptoms the patient describes to you during the interview. The presence of multiple diseases may be the result of any of these circumstances:

☐ Parallel development of different diseases. Both osteoarthritis and gout are separate diseases of older age, and both cause joint pain.

☐ Several illnesses are expressions of a common disease. For example, hyperparathyroidism may be manifested by hypertension, peptic ulcer, and kidney stones, each of which may be treated as a separate condition without recognition of the underlying pathology.

☐ One disease is a complication of another. Coronary artery disease and serious retinal disease (diabetic retinopathy) often are complications of diabetes mellitus.

☐ One disease predisposes to another. For example, a patient with epilepsy may sustain a fracture from falling during a seizure, or a woman may become depressed after breast removal for cancer.

☐ The treatment of one condition gives rise to another. For example, chlorpromazine (Thorazine) may cause an illness resembling hepatitis. As medications and other forms of treatment become more potent, so do their side effects. Conditions arising from treatment (iatrogenic) are increasingly important causes of hospitalization (Steel et al, 1981).

At this point it would be nice to have a precise understanding of exactly what is meant by *disease*. For example, is not diabetic retinopathy really a late-appearing component of diabetes mellitus, rather than a complication? At a practical level, however, an illness with symptoms and therapy distinct from the primary condition can be considered a separate disease.

There is no easy answer to recognizing when the patient's Present Illness is made up of manifestations of two different diseases. Experienced clinicians anticipate complications of common diseases like diabetes mellitus and the side effects of drugs and other therapies. Pattern recognition plays a role in identifying multiple diseases. Finally, when distinct, well-documented symptoms and physical findings cannot be explained by a single diagnosis, multiple diagnoses must be considered (although a great temptation exists to somehow force everything into a single diagnosis).

☐ Psychiatric Diagnosis By Exclusion

Sometimes a patient's illness just doesn't seem to fit any diagnosis. The history may suggest one condition, but the physical findings or laboratory data fail to confirm the initial diagnosis. A frequent but regrettable way out of this frustrating situation is to make an unflattering psychiatric diagnosis by exclusion, saying, in effect, "Nothing in the physical examination or laboratory testing indicates disease, therefore the condition must be 'mental.'"

Sometimes this conclusion is correct; the patient's condition is "mental," but a mental condition with findings just as specific as any traditional bodily disease. The most common of the mental conditions that simulate organic disease is the conversion reaction. The diagnosis is not made by "ruling out everything else," it is made on specific, objective criteria, as illustrated by the following case:

A 38-year-old man came to the emergency room because of retrosternal chest pain suggestive of a myocardial infarction. The EKG was normal, as it may be in the early stages of a coronary artery occlusion, but the ER physician was sufficiently concerned about the patient's history that the man was admitted to the hospital for further observation.

After admission, a detailed interview brought out the fact that exactly one year previously the patient's father had died of lung cancer associated with chest pain strikingly similar to the patient's. Discussion of the son's relationship with his father indicated that the father was a domineering, often brutal man, who the son so hated that he contemplated murder, fantasizing that he would shoot him in the chest. Before the son could act out his impulse (perhaps he would never have done so, for although he had purchased a gun, he also had some genuine feeling of affection for the father, and the family was one in which religion played a role) the father became ill with lung cancer and died shortly afterward, suffering considerable chest pain before his death. The son subsequently felt intense guilt about his father's death, as if his wish had actually brought on the painful cancer.

An additional aspect of the son's illness was that he seemed totally free of anxiety about his condition despite voicing concern about having a "heart attack." The patient remained in the hospital long enough for evidence of a myocardial infarction (cardiac enzymes or EKG changes) to become evident, but all tests remained normal. However, the patient clearly met the major criteria for a conversion reaction: a strong hostile wish that conflicts with personal or social values, identification with his father (one way to atone for guilt of this kind is to impose on oneself the same suffering as wished upon the victim), the anniversary phenomena, and the indifference (la belle indifference), are all objective data that fulfill the criteria by which conversion reactions are diagnosed (Engel, 1983).

Cases like these in which psychological factors are somatized are troubling. Such patients often lead physicians to undertake expensive, prolonged, and sometimes dangerous diagnostic procedures out of fear of "missing something" (discussed in the next chapter), when a more careful interview would establish the basis for the patient's illness as a conversion reaction or other psychological diagnosis. To simply say, "Well, the EKG and enzymes are negative, so it must be psychological" is not valid diagnostic reasoning, and labeling such patients as "mental" is hurtful and bad medical practice.

☐ Therapeutic Trial

Treatment itself can be a diagnostic method. When you finish evaluating your patient, you prescribe the treatment that is most appropriate for the diagnosis. If the patient gets better, you assume the improvement is the result of therapy, thus confirming your initial diagnostic impression. If the patient is not better, or worse, you may conclude your initial diagnosis is wrong and you must then decide about further diagnostic tests.

A *therapeutic trial* is undertaken when you cannot decide among several different diagnoses. You provide the patient with therapy that is specific for only one of the possibilities; if the patient improves, the positive response confirms the diagnosis on which the treatment is based. The process is filled with fallacies: the patient might have improved about the time the treatment is started anyway, or the improvement may be linked to a placebo effect. Further, the wrong therapy may worsen the patient's condition. In some cases, however, a therapeutic trail convincingly establishes the correct diagnosis.

☐ Culture and Geography

The diagnostic aspects of the interview presented in this book have limitations. Inherent in this approach are assumptions about disease probabilities, geography, and culture. For example, if you were interviewing a patient from Alaska who complains of fever and chills, you would probably not think of malaria; if you were in the tropics you would consider malaria from the onset. Similarly, sickle-cell disease in a white person with anemia is so rare it isn't even listed in the differential diagnosis; in black people, however, you would routinely perform a sickle-cell test. Diabetes mellitus is so common among the Papago and Pima Indians of Arizona that Indian Health Service physicians routinely look for the disease; in the Anglo population diabetes is less frequent, and the index of suspecion is lower among physicians serving non-Indian patients. While probabilities are not in themselves diagnostic, they have an important influence on diagnostic thinking.

A man in his fifties who lives in upper New York State spends several months each year in southern Arizona. Because the patient is a heavy smoker, his physician obtains a yearly chest X-ray. When his screening X-ray revealed a discrete nodule not present the year before, the patient was referred to a group of physicians specializing in lung diseases. Several of the group's physicians talked with the patient and examined the X-ray. A battery of tests, including tests for tuberculosis, were negative. Because of the possibility of an early, and possibly curable, lung cancer, major lung surgery was strongly recommended and accepted by the patient.

The lobe of the lung containing the lesion was removed and sent to the pathology laboratory for tissue diagnosis. Microscopic examination revealed *coccidioidomycosis* (Valley Fever), a benign pulmonary condition found only in the desert areas of Arizona and adjacent areas. Valley Fever is so common in Arizona that it accounts for most of the solitary nodules found on X-ray. The New York physicians never considered the condition in their differential diagnosis. A diagnostic bias is understandable in instances like this. Perhaps a detailed interview would have uncovered the fact that the patient spent part of each year in Arizona, but even then the correct diagnosis may not have come to mind.

□ Computers, Diagnosis, and Human Limitations

Although the diagnostic process is a skill that can be understood and, with experience, mastered, when thinking diagnostically we often oversimplify the situation to keep the variables within manageable limits. As more is learned about diseases and as diagnostic criteria are refined, the unaided mind will be unable to cope with the information management skills necessary for accurate diagnosis. The computer will be needed to process large amounts of data and complex diagnostic formulas. The computer may also be the best insurance against diagnostic errors caused by bias, as in the case of the man with Valley Fever. The role of the computer in the interview process is discussed in *Unit VII: Technical Supports.*

□ A Concluding Thought

Finally, every intellectually honest clinician knows that modern medicine's knowledge of disease, although impressive, is still severely limited. Some patients defy diagnosis by the most senior of experienced clinicians, and will probably defy the best efforts of the most powerful computers. Fortunately, nature heals many diseases whether they are diagnosed or not. A vast amount remains to be learned about familiar diseases, and altogether new disease concepts will certainly be identified.

□ REFERENCES AND READINGS

Blois M: The physician's personal workstation. M. D. Computing 1985;2:22–26.
Bursztajn H, Feinbloom R, Hamm RM, et al: Medical Choices, Medical Chances. New York, Dell/ Seymour Lawrence, 1981.

Engel GL: Conversion symptoms. *In* Blacklow RS (ed): MacBryde's Signs and Symptoms, ed 6. Philadelphia, JB Lippincott, 1983, Ch 30.

Ford CV, Polks DG: Conversion disorders: An overview. Psychosomatics 1985;26:371–372.

Feinstein AR: Clinical Judgment. Baltimore, Williams & Wilkins, 1967.

Fulginiti VA: Pediatric Clinical Problem Solving. Baltimore, Williams & Wilkins, 1981, pp 47–54.

Klass P: Camels, zebras, and fascinomas. Discover 1985; March:44–46.

Roueche B: The Medical Detectives—II. New York, Time Books, 1984, pp. 345–358.

Rund DA: Problem Solving. *In* Taylor RB (ed): Family Medicine: Principles and Practice, ed 2. New York, Springer-Verlag, 1983, pp 321–335.

Steel K, Gertman PM, et al: Iatrogenic illness on a general medical service at a university hospital. N Engl J Med 1981; 304:638–642.

Wulff HR: Rational Diagnosis and Treatment, ed 2. London, Blackwell Scientific Publications, 1981.

Ziporyn T: Medical decision making: Analyzing options in the face of uncertainty. JAMA 1983;249:2133–2142.

Uncertainty: A Fact of Life
Do Something!
Appeal to Authority
Share Your Uncertainty With
  the Patient?
Uncertainty and Interviewing

CHAPTER 11

UNCERTAINTY IN PROBLEM-SOLVING

☐ Uncertainty: A Fact of Life

The goal of the diagnostic process, in any of its strategies, is to reduce uncertainty. As you interview and examine a patient, many possible diagnoses (either at the *organ/system* or disease level) are eliminated, and fewer remain for further consideration. Often the diagnostic alternatives are similar enough that there is no practical consequence in terms of treatment, but sometimes a correct diagnosis is crucial—for example, deciding whether a patient's chest pain is caused by a benign inflammation of the chest wall muscles, or results from a potentially fatal narrowing of the coronary arteries. Even after a careful interview, physical examination, and laboratory testing, a degree of diagnostic fuzziness often remains.

Uncertainty is a fundamental fact of the health care process, and is particularly difficult to live with during your student years. Dr. Donald G. Anderson, a former dean of the University of Rochester School of Medicine and Dentistry, comments:

> Very little of all we know about health and disease is known with completeness or certainty. Many students enter medical school expecting that medical science has developed a body of knowledge which, if learned with diligence, will enable a physician to practice with confidence and competence. That important judgments and decisions must frequently be made on the basis of fragmentary knowledge is a discovery for which many students are ill prepared intellectually or emotionally.
>
> Accepting uncertainty, and dealing with it effectively, is for many students the most difficult adjustment they must make in medical school. Some, to their own unhappiness and that of their future patients, never succeed in making it.

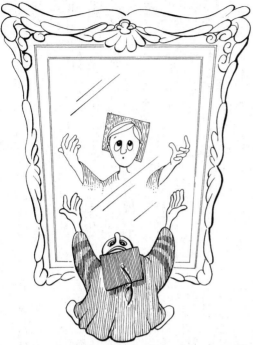

*"Mirror, mirror on the wall
please tell me I know it all !"*

The psychological pressure to achieve certainty is a source of clinical errors. Ingenious research into the psychology of decision making demonstrates that our need to eliminate the anxiety of uncertainty sometimes dupes us into choices that an objective analysis indicates are not the best ones (Kahneman and Tversky, 1982). For example, physicians may recommend, and patients accept, a diagnostic procedure whose risk is greater than the condition under consideration (for example, doing risky surgery to rule out the slight chance that a tumor is cancerous). How a question is phrased makes a difference in the choice made—people will choose a procedure with a 90 per cent survival rate but reject one with a 10 per cent mortality.

Unfortunately, the medical education process, with its covert pressures to achieve error-free performance, does not reward uncertainty; rather, it encourages compulsiveness that drives the physician to

...."run the extra mile" and rule out the rare disease entity that a less conscientious person might fail to consider... (and) to check and double-check laboratory data and physical findings for minute changes that might be of significance ... traits that are socially valuable but personally expensive.

(Gabbard, 1985).

Once you accept the fact that often you will have to act on the basis of partial knowledge, you will minimize the effects of uncertainty.

□ Do Something!

At the basis of much of our decision making is a deep-seated belief that *any* loss is blameworthy and avoidable, and will result in guilt, censure by colleagues, and maybe a devastating malpractice suit. "Doing something" is the most common response to these concerns. Doing something gives us, and our patients, a sense of confidence and control, whereas doing nothing somehow implies professional ignorance or failure.

The story is told about a patient who saw a physician for a lingering problem. The physician recommended surgery. The patient sought a second opinion from a well known surgeon. After a careful interview and examination, the consultant told the patient that he felt sure the condition was self-limiting, and he saw no need for surgery.
Several weeks later the patient received a $200 bill for the second opinion. The patient returned the bill unpaid, with a note saying, in effect, "For doing nothing you charge me $200?"
The surgeon then sent a new bill, as follows:
> For doing nothing................... *No charge*
> For knowing to do nothing.............. $200

In many situations, the body or mind, given a chance may cure itself. Just the decision to seek a physician's help starts in motion behaviors that cure. The initial interview and examination are powerful placebos, a fact often overlooked since therapy is so often prescribed on the first visit, even if not clearly indicated. Also, some diagnostic tests, and most therapies, involve both risks and substantial costs. Mold (1986) describes a clinical "cascade effect," a chain of interlocking procedures, starting with some minor abnormality or concern that triggers a clinician's anxiety, which exposes patients to escalating risks. Spiro (1985) suggests that sometimes it is reasonable to treat a patient despite diagnostic uncertainty:

Physicians have been trained to think of themselves as scientists; they have learned to search for a biologically detectable reason for every complaint. Partly they do so in the fear that they may be sued for missing something. Partly, I suspect, they follow every clue because that is what they have been taught to do in medical school and that is what they have been praised for during residency training....

Why not treat indigestion wih the currently effective drugs and wait ten days or so to see what happens before embarking on the long diagnostic work-up? Most (patients) were frightened at the thought that *their* physician would not immediately try to pinpoint the physical cause of every complaint, regardless of cost.... They want every study to be done as soon as possible and do not care about the cost.

Physicians often are uncomfortable with this philosophy: it clashes with the image of the doctor as a person of action. Patients, too, often want something done (although as a result of patient education activities, many accept a conservative approach). Thus, the quest for certitude, no matter what the monetary and psychological costs, distorts medical practice.

☐ Appeal to Authority

Another way to calm one's anxieties about uncertainty is to depend to an excessive degree on advice from experienced physicians. Or we may consult authoritative books. Both approaches have their place, but also their weaknesses. We may let our initial impressions limit our reading or advice seeking in such a way that new alternatives will not come to light. And it is easy to believe that partial knowledge is complete knowledge—it is difficult to identify the omissions and limits of that knowledge.

☐ Share Your Uncertainty With the Patient?

Despite uncertainty being a normal, natural part of the health care process, physicians often want to appear to their patients and their colleagues to be decisive and self-confident. Students, especially, feel vulnerable and have an understandable wish to appear to their patients as experienced clinicians. Usually, however, the true state of affairs is revealed with qualifying phrases such as "I think . . ." or "It is probably . . . ," or by nonverbal behaviors that indicate lack of confidence in whatever is said. Far better is to remind the patient, and yourself, that you are a medical student, and also that the interview is only the beginning of the diagnostic process. (In any event, communicating a diagnosis to the patient is the responsibility of the attending physician unless specifically delegated to you.)

Sharing your uncertainty with the patient can go too far, however, especially about serious but extremely rare diagnoses. Sometimes this kind of message is given to the patient:

"Mr. Smith, my examination tells me that all your symptoms can be accounted for by a cataract. I don't find any evidence of a tumor of the eye, which, while remotely possible, is extremely unlikely."

Why raise the possibility of a tumor if it is so unlikely that nothing in the way of further examination is planned? Statements like this are often unconsciously motivated by the wish to appear to be an astute diagnostician or to have thought of "everything" should a serious condition actually be discovered. There may even be the thought that if something rare but serious escapes detection and the patient later sues the doctor, the record would show that the possibility had been considered from the beginning, and the patient told about it. The recital of remotely possible diagnoses usually is made quickly, almost as an afterthought, and often with a lot of medical jargon. What this kind of sharing usually accomplishes is confusion and unnecessary worry. Of course, when your initial impression suggests that something serious may well be present and that further testing is warranted, giving false reassurance is neither honest nor helpful.

□ Uncertainty and Interviewing

Early in the interview, usually during the Present Illness, you realize that you haven't a good idea of the diagnosis. A common response is to repeatedly go over the same material—to examine the same symptoms over and over in the hope that buried in some minute detail is the key to everything. Often, the added information obscures rather than clarifies, and wastes valuable time. The best advice that can be given is this: obtain a broad overview of the entire history—the *Fundamental Four*—before narrowing in on a specific area. Occasionally the answer does lie in a microanalysis of some small aspect of the patient's history, but knowing where to probe for details can be achieved only after you have had a chance to survey the overall history.

□ Conclusion

Certainty cannot be achieved in medical care, and attempts to achieve it increase the risk and expense to the patient. The reading list below cites a variety of readable books and articles that explore this topic in more detail.

□ REFERENCES AND READINGS

Allman RM, Steinberg EP, et al: Physician tolerance for uncertainty. Use of liver-spleen scans to detect metastasis. JAMA 1985; 254:246–248.

Allman WF: Staying alive in the 20th century. Science 85, 1985; October, pp 31–37.

Bursztajn H, Feinbloom R, Hamm RM, et al: Medical Choices, Medical Chances, New York, Dell/Seymour Lawrence, 1981.

Froom J, Feinbloom R, Mellvile RG: Risks of referral. J Fam Pract 1984; 18:623–626.

Gabbard GO: The role of compulsiveness in the normal physician. JAMA 1985; 254:2926–2929.

Haney CA: Psychosocial factors involved in medical decision making. In Coombs RH, Vincent CE (eds): Psychosocial Aspects of Medical Training, Springfield, IL, Charles C Thomas, 1971, pp. 404–425.

Herwig TT: "I don't know." JAMA 1986; 256:2348.

Kahneman D, Tversky A: The psychology of preferences. Sci Am 1982; January, pp 160–173.

Katz J: Acknowledging uncertainty. In The Silent World of Doctor and Patient. New York, The Free Press/Macmillan, 1984, chap VII.

Knight J: Developing tolerance for uncertainty. In: Doctor-To-Be. New York, Appleton-Century-Crofts, 1981, chap 9.

McKean K: Decisions, decisions. Discover 1985; June, pp 22–31.

Mold JW, Stein HF: The cascade effect in the clinical care of patients. N Engl J Med 1986; 314:512–514. Also, see Correspondence, N Engl J Med 1986; 315:319–320.

Schwartz WB: Decision analysis: A look at the chief complaints. N Engl J Med 1979; 300:556–589.

Spiro HM: Delayed diagnosis of disease. JAMA 1985; 253:2258.

Weinstein MD, Feinberg HV: Clinical Decision Analysis. Philadelphia, WB Saunders Co, 1980.

Ziporyn T: Medical decision making: Analyzing options in the face of uncertainty. JAMA 1983; 249:2133–2142.

UNIT III

HEALTH PROMOTION

CHAPTER 12

THE HEALTH PROMOTION INTERVIEW

Thus far, the interview has been discussed in the context of clinical problem-solving. The other major focus of the interview is *Health Promotion* or *Health Maintenance*. In such situations the patient feels well. The visit to a physician may be a required part of an insurance or job application, or the patient may be motivated by an awareness of the value of detecting illness or health risks early and of adopting a healthy lifestyle. Health Promotion is a rapidly growing area of medical practice, and has already accounted for gains in the health of many segments of society. For example, immunizations have eliminated many of the serious infectious diseases, the Pap test has made cervical cancer a rarity, and the incidence of myocardial infarction (heart attack) has reversed its upward trend as a result of changes in patients' diet, smoking, and exercise patterns. While curative medicine will continue to increase life span, major gains in overall health will result from more effective health promotion activities.

☐ Objectives

The objectives of a Health Promotion History are:
1. Early detection of disease.
2. Prevention of disease by reducing or eliminating risk factors.
3. Establishing a baseline of data for the future.

In contrast to the focused Problem-Centered interview, the Health Promotion interview is a complete inventory of current physical and mental functioning, plus a complete listing of the patient's Past Medical History, Family Medical History, and Personal/Social (Life Style) History. The Health Promotion interview, which focuses on health, complements the Problem-Centered interview, which focuses on illness.

Note that the Health Promotion database consists of the *same information categories,* the *Fundamental Four,* as the Problem-Centered interview; however, each category is explored in greater detail.

The Present Illness might better be described as an *inventory of current health.* It consists of a complete Review of Systems (ROS). You ask the patient about a large number of common symptoms in every system of the body. The objective of this review is identifying symptoms that may signal early but significant disease. In a sense, you are examining the patient by the use of words rather than physical examination techniques.

The Past Health History focuses on significant past illnesses which have implications for the future. This history alerts you to conditions that can reappear (such as a peptic ulcer or a previously treated cancer), or diseases that cannot recur (such as appendicitis in a patient who had an appendectomy). You also ask about current medications and medication sensitivities, immunizations, and chronic illnesses that may influence management of any new problem. Diabetes mellitus, for example, influences management of medical problems unrelated to the diabetes, and a history of a penicillin reaction will influence your choice of medications when treating any infection.

Family Health History (Hereditary/Contagious History) establishes the existence of disease in blood relatives (parents, grandparents, brothers, sisters, children of the patient), and also the health of spouse and close associates. This information alerts you to hereditary disease (for example, cystic fibrosis) or contagious disease (such as tuberculosis) which may influence the future health of your patient and the patient's family and for which you can take preventive measures. "Family Health History" is really not an accurate term unless you include all persons who form the patient's close social environment. Patients may contract *contagious* diseases from persons who are not family members in the strict sense.

The *Personal/Social History* (Lifestyle) includes *social relationships* in and out of the family, occupational influences, and personal habits such as poor diet, alcohol intake, and smoking, which are health risks, or which may influence medical management. Recreation, travel, financial situation (ability to afford basic necessities, including health insurance), "significant others," sexual preferences and practices, and spiritual beliefs all have implications for physical and mental health.

The following examples demonstrate how information obtained during a Health Promotion interview is of practical value in prevention or early detection of disease, or in establishing a baseline for future use.

□ Early Detection of Disease

An older man in the hospital for an elective hernia repair mentioned "leg cramps" during the routine Circulatory System Review. He considered these a part of old age, not indicative of a disease ("You expect a few aches and pains at my age."), and had never consulted a physician about it. Physical examination clearly demonstrated the presence of significant arterial disease for which effective therapy was available, and which, if left untreated, could progress to incapacitating vascular insufficiency.

A middle-aged housewife, during an initial health evaluation with a new physician, said that she felt quite well, but routine questioning indicated the presence of weight loss, constipation, and sleep disturbance. Her physician recognized that these rather common minor complaints, taken together, suggested the existence of a significant though unrecognized depression. Further questioning brought out the fact that a family business was not doing well and that the patient was more concerned than she was willing to admit. Brief psychotherapy redirected her depression into constructive action.

A woman in her 50's has a strong family history of breast cancer. When a breast cancer detection program was announced in her community she enrolled. On her initial examination a small mass was felt, and a mammogram confirmed the presence of a suspicious lesion. A biopsy was positive for cancer: minimal breast surgery completely removed the growth, and the patient has been free of cancer for five years.

□ Prevention

During a routine insurance examination, a patient mentioned that he had had "rheumatism" as a child. Although the patient currently felt entirely well, the clinician, alerted by the history, discovered a faint but definite heart murmur, the result of childhood rheumatic fever. Thorough cardiac evaluation revealed definite heart valve disease for which prophylactic medication is mandatory to avoid complications.

A young mother indicated to her physician that she never wore seat belts while driving and had not thought about obtaining a restraint for her young daughter. The physician's clinic had a program for loaning infant restraint seats to their patients, and the patient accepted one. She also started wearing her seat belt while driving. Several months later the patient's car was involved in a major accident. Neither mother nor child received significant injury.

A 35-year-old motorcyclist hasn't had a tetanus booster since childhood *and doesn't wear a helmet. A moment's discussion of the need for both may save the patient from serious illness or permanent disability later on.*

An excellent way to develop a sensitivity to practical preventive medicine is to ask yourself, "Could this illness have been prevented?" whenever you see someone with a serious illness. For example, had a patient admitted to the hospital with pneumonia ever been offered the pneumococcal vaccine? Would wearing a seat belt have prevented serious injury in an automobile accident? Could simple dietary advice have reduced the risk for a patient with a heart attack or hypertension? Could a few home precautions have prevented a child's accidental poisoning or an elderly person's fall?

☐ Baseline

A 23-year-old woman made an appointment with her physician because she believed she was three or four months pregnant. Her blood pressure was 140/85 and she had frequent headaches. The only time she had seen her physician was for a Health Promotion examination when she first moved to town 18 months before. The blood pressure at that time was 100/70, and she rarely had headaches. The new blood pressure, compared to the baseline reading, indicated definite hypertension. (Even though 140/85 is within the normal adult range, the amount of change, 40/15, was a significant alteration from normal and consistent with pre-eclampsia, a potentially serious pregnancy-related condition.) The patient's Family Health History included mild hypertension in both parents, a risk factor that added to the significance of the rise in blood pressure.

☐ Treatment and Patient Education

When people are ill and uncomfortable, they are usually willing to undergo treatment. When they feel well, prevention of illness or treatment of asymptomatic disease is often resisted. Despite the proven effectiveness of seat belts in reducing death and injury from automobile accidents, people resist their routine use. When an element of addiction is present, such as with smoking, changing life style is difficult, even if the patient is intellectually convinced of the danger to health. It is in these areas that the medical profession faces some of its greatest challenges. Unfortunately, the fields of Preventive Medicine and Public Health lack the drama of the curative specialties, and fail to attract the interest and support they deserve.

Prevention is also a part of treatment of some conditions, and was discussed in *Chapter 9: The Problem-Centered Interview.*

□ Practical Health Promotion Strategies

Although many people are health conscious and seek out health promotion care, others are unwilling to undergo the time and expense of a complete *Health Promotion* evaluation. Fortunately, a variety of approaches support health promotion. Health promotion can be incorporated into problem-centered care, as explained in the next chapter. Questionnaires and computers, discussed in the last section of this book, are inexpensive but effective substitutes for expensive health care personnel. Large automated multiphasic health testing programs, using "mass production" methods of history taking and examination capable of screening large numbers of persons, have been claimed to be effective, as have smaller programs in corporations and other specialized settings. In some instances, a few questions can identify persons at risk for certain conditions.

Finally, groups at high risk for specific diseases can be identified and appropriate measures taken. For example, hospital personnel at risk for getting hepatitis can be immunized with appropriate hepatitis vaccines, and screening of Jews whose families came from Eastern Europe can detect Tay-Sachs disease. The knowledge of risk factors, discussed in *Chapter 8: Risk Factors in Diagnosis and Treatment,* will help you provide your patients with an appropriate health promotion program.

□ The Premarital Examination

The premarital examination illustrates many of the principles of health promotion, and addresses so many problems of contemporary society that it deserves special consideration. Society's high rate of troubled and failing marriages and the epidemic of domestic violence and abuse involving both children and adults suggest that marriage and family living is no simple matter, yet it is easier to get a marriage license than a driver's license. The premarital examination offers an exceptional opportunity for health promotion.

The premarital examination is more than a time for providing accurate sexual information. The couple about to marry should be questioned about *genetic diseases.* Not everyone who has a family history of a serious genetic disease understands the risks of having children with the same condition. A human tragedy can be avoided with no more than five minutes' inquiry into the Family Medical History. Another simple step that will prevent some birth defects is ensuring that women are immune to rubella (German measles). *Genital abnormalities* that may prevent satisfactory sexual activity and becoming pregnant are detected during a physical examination, which should be a part of the premarital evaluation. Information about *family planning* should be offered to persons about to marry. Don't assume that everyone understands the available contraception options. Preliminary discussion about what *parent-*

ing is all about may prevent instances of child abuse later on and open the door to a healthier family life than would otherwise be the case. Advice about obtaining adequate health insurance may prevent costly financial stress later. Incorporating a meaningful premarital examination into your practice can be the first link in a long-term, satisfying professional relationship.

☐ REFERENCES AND READINGS

Frame P: A critical review of adult health maintenance (4 pts). J Fam Pract 1986;22 (April–July):341–346, 417–422, 511–519; vol 23: 29–39.

Johnson TA Jr, Eakin KM: Health maintenance and screening. *In* Taylor RB (ed); Family Medicine: Principles and Practice, ed 2. New York, Springer-Verlag, 1983, pp 295–313.

Payton CE: Sexual Counseling. *In* Taylor RB (ed): Family Medicine: Principles and Practice, ed 2. New York, Springer-Verlag, 1983, pp 219–236.

CHAPTER 13

A COMBINED PROBLEM-CENTERED/HEALTH PROMOTION INTERVIEW

When seeing an ill patient, your first priority is obtaining a *Problem-Centered* history. *Health Promotion* questions are saved for later in the interview, or for a subsequent visit. The experienced interviewer knows what is relevant to the immediate problem, and what can safely be deferred. As a student, you will have to decide whether to attempt a Problem-Centered history, with its decisions about what is relevant, the first time you interview a new patient. The alternative is to do a *complete* history, and afterwards separate the Problem-Centered information from the Health Promotion information.

If you already have some clinical background, you will probably have little trouble doing a Problem-Centered interview first, and then rounding out the interview with Health Promotion information. You'll find the "Think Organs/Systems" approach presented in this book a help in maintaining your perspective, even if you don't know a lot about specific diseases.

If you are a total stranger to clinical medicine, you may feel more secure doing a complete history at the onset of your training. I do urge, however, that you make the change to the Problem-Centered format early. Otherwise, you may find the habit of doing a complete history has become so ingrained that you'll have trouble breaking away when you are no longer able to spend an hour or more doing an interview. You may find yourself asking 80-year-old patients if they had the usual childhood illnesses like measles, German measles, mumps, and chickenpox. (Would it make any practical difference in caring for the patient?) You may also get into the habit of asking other "routine questions" that make little sense to the patient.

The essential difference between the Problem-Centered history and the Health Promotion history is the *degree* to which the data in each category are collected. The same *Fundamental Four* categories of clinical information form the framework for both types of clinical activities. In a Problem-Centered interview you are guided by the principle of relevance: you focus on those facts of the patient's health history that are helpful in solving the patient's problem. In a Health Promotion interview you cast a wider net to capture information that detects early illness, highlights preventive measures for the patient to consider, and records a set of baseline measurements as a reference for the future.

You should complete a comprehensive history (Problem-Centered plus Health Promotion History) early in any continuing clinical relationship. Sometimes you will discover an unexpected co-existing condition. You may, for example, discover a history of significant rectal bleeding in a patient admitted to the hospital for treatment of an unrelated condition. Also, a comprehensive history helps you appreciate the medical, psychological, and social context that will influence treatment of the immediate problem—for example, pre-existing diabetes in a patient admitted with myocardial infarction, or the existence of depression that may interfere with a patient's cooperation in the treatment of a peptic ulcer. Preventive medicine services, such as updating immunizations or patient education, are easy to accomplish in the hospital, and with hospital care costing hundreds of dollars a day, the patient should receive every possible service that contributes to comprehensive care. Unfortunately, hospital staffs are so focused on acute care that the possibility of adding health maintenance services is often overlooked.

There are several advantages to mastering a Problem-Centered interview at the beginning of your training:

- ☐ You will not have to learn a new approach later on when the time constraints of practice dictate Problem-Centered interviewing.
- ☐ Ill persons may not tolerate, physically or emotionally, a complete interview when first seen for interview and physical examination. Their physical endurance may be limited, and they may become impatient if the discussion involves matters of little or no *immediate* relevance.
- ☐ Time is often a realistic factor. Patients you see in an outpatient setting may not be prepared to spend the amount of time needed for a complete evaluation. Hospitalized patients appear to have plenty of time for a complete history, but this is not always so. Your interview may be interrupted so that the patient can go to the X-ray department or receive treatment. Better to have a complete, although brief, Problem-Centered history than an incomplete comprehensive history.
- ☐ Since much of a patient's total history is reviewed while doing a Problem-Centered history, often it is relatively easy to complete the history by adding the remaining information.
- ☐ Sometimes the first answer a patient gives to a question may not be accurate or complete. Patients start thinking about some topics only after you have moved on to something else, and wish they had given

a different or more complete answer. By performing a Problem-Centered interview first and then reviewing the health history from the Health Promotion perspective, the patient may add information that is relevant to the immediate problem. (The patient has other opportunities to add information at the end of the interview when you ask, "Is there anything else you want to add?" and during the physical examination when examining regions of the body reminds patients of things they had not thought about during the interview.) Knowing that you'll have a second chance to go over the *Fundamental Four* areas of information gives you the security you need to move from one major area of information to the next. Getting lost in a mass of detail happens in both types of interviews, but a time-limited Problem-Centered interview forces you to get the *overall picture*.

These advantages may not be enough to overcome one great disadvantage of this two-tiered approach: knowing what is relevant and what is not. If you lose your way and cannot develop a coherent Problem-Centered history, you'll come away feeling defeated, and the patient may wonder what was going on. At least with the comprehensive history, you can't get lost (well, you can, but not easily).

You'll have opportunities to try both approaches and decide which is best for you. Perhaps you will use one approach in some settings and the other in other settings. Observe experienced physicians and their styles. With time you will settle on techniques that are best for you.

UNIT IV

COMMUNICATION TECHNIQUES

14

VERBAL (SPOKEN) TECHNIQUES

Communication is the heart of the interview. The nature of communication is not easy to describe (an attempt is made in the concluding section of this chapter), but for the purposes of this book, communication takes place when physician and patient *share information*. Most of this information is communicated by spoken words (verbal communication) and nonverbal communication. This chapter discusses the uses and properties of spoken communication; nonverbal communication is discussed in the next chapter. (These two kinds of communication are intimately interrelated; separating them is artificial but necessary for discussion.)

Spoken communication, from the interviewer's perspective, serves three major purposes in the clinical interview

1. Establishing rapport.
2. Getting information from the patient.
3. Giving information to the patient.

Rapport has already been discussed in *Chapter 4*, which you may want to review now.

☐ Getting Information

A major task of the clinical interview is diagnosis—the naming of the disease causing an illness for which the patient seeks your help. Diagnosis also includes identifying the patient's emotions and attitudes that accompany the illness.

Questioning is the major information-getting technique. There are three major types of questions used in an interview.

1. Open-ended.

2. Limited choice.
3. Yes/No.

Clarification and *elaboration* are two secondary kinds of questions.

Open-ended questions announce an area of interest. They do not suggest either the content or the structure of the answer. In effect, to any broad area of interest, the interviewer is saying, "I'm interested, please go on." To initiate the interview, for example, you might ask, "Why have you come to the clinic today?" or "How can I be of help?" Whatever the answer, resist the temptation to immediately focus on details of the *Sacred Seven* or *Fundamental Four*. Instead, remain open to what the patient wants to talk about by replying, "Tell me more about it." This unstructured response spreads the widest possible net by indicating to the patient, "Tell me as much as you want, in any way you like, about. . ." whatever topic is under discussion. If a patient says the problem is, "Back pain," a open-ended response would be, "Tell me more about it," or perhaps just repeating (with a questioning voice), "Back pain?"

The open-ended question is much more than an interviewing technique; it reflects an open, inquisitive *attitude* towards each patient. It stands in contrast to an outlook that seems to say, "I've seen everything; just tell me in a word or two what your problem is, and I'll take it from there," followed by a rapid-fire effort to "get the facts." But what are the facts—how do you as interviewer know where to look unless the patient tells you? No physician, however experienced, can accurately anticipate the uniqueness of each human being. Consider how a "forget the open-ended stuff, just get the facts" attitude would have been far off target in this instance:

The patient, a 45-year-old man, when asked about the reason for the office visit, said simply, "Stomach pain." The interviewer said, "Tell me more about it." The patient then said that he had recently lost his job, his wife had left him, and the bank had foreclosed on his house. He was living alone in a small apartment, eating poorly and had started to drink.

His primary problem was depression. The abdominal pain, which was nothing more serious than gastritis, disappeared as he started to get his life in order. Had the interviewer immediately followed the statement of the initial complaint of stomach pain by asking for specific descriptive information—*the Sacred Seven*—the essence of his problem might have been missed. An expensive and inconclusive medical evaluation of abdominal pain would have been pursued, with mounting costs, equivocal results, and trials of powerful medications. Sadly, patients like this even undergo exploratory surgery for abdominal disease that doesn't exist because the clinician's perspective of the patient was too limited.

Open-ended questions have another virtue; they quickly cover an area of the patient's history. A single question about Past Medical History, "How has your health been in the past?" may produce more relevant information than dozens of specific questions. Sometimes you want to quickly cover an area of health history which you doubt will be productive, but which you don't want to omit altogether. In the Review of Systems, for example, a single open-ended question such as, "How are your bones, muscles and joints?" or "How are your eyes and vision?" may yield unanticipated information.

Open-ended techniques have important limitations. For one thing, many persons do not think in generalities. "How has your health been?" or "Tell me more about it" may just bring you a puzzled look. Also, in *every* interview you need to ask about important factual details. The best interview is an appropriate blend of the techniques described in this chapter. The open-ended technique, however, often is omitted altogether in the desire to deal as quickly as possible with specifics. Sometimes the long way around is the shortest way home. Try out this technique and find when it is useful. When it does work, it takes you quickly to the heart of the matter.

Limited choice questions are focused; they ask the patient to supply a limited item of information.

"How old are you?"

"What did the pain feel like?"

"What medicines are you taking?"

"What past illnesses have you had?"

Either/Or (a type of limited choice) questions restrict the patient to just two choices, and are best avoided unless you are certain no other possibilities exist.

"Did the pain go to your neck or your back?"

"Did you take codeine or Demerol when the pain started?"

Yes/No questions are just that: the patient is asked no more than the presence or absence of some bit of information.

"Do you have fever?"

"Did you vomit?"

"Have you had appendicitis?"

"Was anyone else sick at home?"

In addition to these three primary question forms are two secondary forms—clarification and elaboration—which ask for more information.

Clarification is a request for the patient to explain or provide more detail about information already stated but that you don't fully understand.

"I'm not clear about what you mean by feeling 'dizzy.' Please explain in more detail."

"Was it before or after eating that the pain started?"

Elaboration is similar but asks the patient to add a new dimension of information to that already given.

"When the dizziness started, what else did you feel?"

"When the argument started, what in addition to money problems was brought up?"

In addition to techniques that ask for facts in various degrees of detail are techniques that *facilitate* or *encourage* the kind of response the patient is already giving. Verbal and nonverbal responses provide intermittent positive reinforcement that sustains the interview.

- □ An occasional smile.
- □ Leaning towards the patient.
- □ Nod of the head.
- □ "That's fine, please continue."
- □ "And then?"
- □ "Uh huh, please go on."

Silence can be a powerful form of encouragement. Sometimes a patient will fall silent and seem lost in thought. (Twenty or thirty seconds of this kind of reverie seem like hours, and you will feel an urge to say something. Patients seem unaware of time, however.) Your nonverbal expressions of interest, and a degree of confidence, are essential if you use silence as a facilitating technique. Discipline yourself to remain quiet until the patient's attention returns; you may be rewarded with important information.

"You really seemed lost in thought just now (or a few minutes ago) when I asked about cancer. Is there something you want to ask about?"

Repeating the patient's last words indicates that you are interested in what has just been said and would like to know more about it.

Patient: "It hurts."

Doctor: *"It hurts?"*

Patient: "I couldn't walk after that."

Doctor: *"Couldn't walk?"*

Patient: "I have been very upset lately."

Doctor: *"Upset?"*

Confirming or acknowledging what the patient has just said indicates you understand thus far and encourages the patient to continue.

Reflection is a response, based on your observation, which points out to the patient feelings:

"When you mentioned your boss just now, you made a fist and really looked angry."

Summarization and *paraphrasing* are more detailed forms of acknowledgement.

"Before we go on, let me summarize what I understand so far. You were feeling well until last evening, when after dinner you became nauseated and felt a dull ache in the right side of your abdomen. Then, about 30 minutes later you vomited, but the pain continued. You took a couple of Tums but that didn't help at all. Is this correct so far?"

A restatement of what the patient has told you gives both you and the patient a chance to correct errors or misunderstandings before going on. During a complicated history, or when dealing with something unfamiliar, summarize frequently. This is also a good time in the interview to make notes, rather than trying to write continuously as the patient talks.

Asking for a description of *a typical day* is a particularly valuable technique to understand the patient as a person, to identify who are the important persons in the patient's life, and to understand the patient's lifestyle.

"Please describe for me a typical day for you—from getting up to going to bed."

"What is an average day like for you?"

You will be amazed at the variety of life patterns that patients consider normal or routine. The insights gained may suggest diagnostic and therapeutic possibilities not possible by any other interviewing technique.

A 45-year-old woman couldn't understand why she felt exhausted. She had no other symptoms of illness, had been exceptionally healthy in the past and could think of nothing in her lifestyle that was stressful.

The answer came when she related her typical day: up at 4:30 a.m. to milk the cows and do farm chores, breakfast at 6:00 a.m. for her husband and five children, then off to work at a nearby factory producing sportswear, home by 5:00 p.m., dinner, ironing, cleaning the house ("I like a neat, clean house"), to bed by 11:00 or 11:30 p.m.

For years this woman had worked this hard as a matter of course. Finally age, perhaps disappointment and menopausal changes were catching up with her.

□ Giving Information

An interview is not just a method of obtaining information; it is also an opportunity for you to give various kinds of information.

Interpretation is a response in which the interviewer offers a generalization encompassing a number of observations.

"It sounds as if you don't like being a medical student."

"Isn't this the same reaction you had last year when visiting your sister?"

Evaluation statements add a dimensions of "good or bad" to what the patient has related.

"That doesn't seem like a very good idea."

"I don't see how anything can go wrong with that approach. Sounds good to me."

Interpretations and evaluations are tricky until you have had a continuing relationship with the patient and feel comfortable about undertaking what amounts to minor, and sometimes not so minor, psychotherapy.

Support and *reassurance* demonstrate your interest, concern and understanding. By indicating that you recognize how the patient feels, you give evidence of your willingness to understand and help. Supportive statements help the patient express feelings and report additional information, thereby strengthening rapport.

"That must have been very painful."

"I can share your feeling of frustration."

"That's a very understandable response to this sort of situation."

Patient education is an important trend in modern health care. In addition to providing information needed for self-care, you promote a sense of partnership with the patient in the health care process. See *Chapter 19: The Interview as Therapy and Patient Education* for more discussion of information-giving in the clinical interview.

□ Directing and Regulating the Interview

□ FOCUSING

Each section of the interview must have direction and control. You will want to cover some topics in more detail than others. Available time and the patient's condition determine the overall structure and content of the interview.

Many of the techniques already described are designed to redirect, clarify, or amplify the patient's initial response. Interrupt the patient who wanders, and refocus attention on relevant material. Some patients have difficulty responding to a specific question. They may digress, or may provide more detail than you need.

> "Let's think just about the question I asked you right now. We can come back to this other matter later."

You may have to tactfully but repeatedly interrupt a patient who is telling you more about a subject than you want to know.

> "You've given me as much information about that as I need for now. Let's move on to. . ."

The *overly talkative* patient is discussed in *Chapter 20: Difficult Relationships.*

□ Transitional Statements

In addition to focusing the patient's attention on some areas and moving past others, you will have to aid the patient in making the transition from one section of the history to the next. You do this with a brief statement summarizing the section just finished, followed by an open-ended inquiry about the next area:

> "I understand about your past health—now I'd like to ask about the health of your family. Are there any illnesses that seem to run in the family?"

> "Now that we have talked about the problem that brought you into the hospital, I'd like to review other aspects of your health to see if there are other conditions that also merit some attention."

If your patient does not see the relevance of a question or an emotionally charged personal/social topic, a brief explanation of the reason for the line of questioning is helpful.

> "Sometimes, Mr. Jones, personal problems can lead to muscle tension and backache. How are things going in your personal life?"

A smooth transition between the Family Medical History and the area of the Personal/Social History detailing the patient's *social relationships* is to ask, "Who is at home?"

In a Health Promotion interview, a single statement mentioning prevention or early detection is usually adequate explanation.

> "Now that we've covered the problem of your back pain, I'd like to review

your overall health to see if there are other problems that might just be starting, or if some simple measures now might prevent problems later.''

Moving from details of one section to an initial open-ended question of the next area provides a smooth transition in all types of interviews. In the ROS, for example:

"How are your ears? (pause); hearing loss? (pause); ringing noises? (pause); discharge? (pause); earaches? (pause) How are your eyes? (pause); blurred vision? (pause); double vision (pause). . . .''

☐ Documenting

Not only do you obtain information from the patient, you need to be sure the information is accurate. Patients forget or misinterpret statements made in the past. You cannot challenge the accuracy of every statement your patient makes, but where you sense inaccuracy, clarification and elaboration are necessary. A patient may say, for example, "I am allergic to penicillin" when only non-specific side effects like nausea or diarrhea occurred. If you question some fact, ask, "What do you mean by 'allergy,' " or "What happened to you when you had the allergy to penicillin?"

Similarly, patients may incorrectly quote clinician's diagnoses. Obtaining past records from previous health providers is frequently an essential part of accurate clinical information gathering. In the future, when medical records are computerized, you will be able to get data from primary documents created at the time the patient actually received care.

Documenting is a facet of the question of patient *reliability* discussed in *Chapter 16: Procedure Basics.*

☐ Ineffective Techniques

Suggestive or leading questions give the patient the answer to the question:

Has the pain gone into your left arm from your chest?

Better: Does the pain go anywhere?

Was the pain worse after a big meal?

Better: Does a big meal affect it?

You haven't had any fever, have you?

Better: Have you had a fever?

What is the pain like—is it sharp?

Better: What was the pain like?

Why questions that ask patients to account for their behavior should be avoided. It is difficult to being a question with "why" and avoid overtones of accusation.

Why didn't you take the medicine?

Better: Was there a problem in taking the medicine?

If you've had the pains for years, why did you wait until now to see a doctor?

Better: Since you say you've had the pains for years, what made you decide to see a doctor now?

Multiple questions leave the patient confused.

Was it on Saturday or Sunday you first noticed the bleeding, and was the blood pinkish, and how much was there?

Better: What day did the bleeding begin? (Answer)
  What color was the blood? (Answer)
  How much blood was there? (Answer)

What I need to know is at what age was the onset, how frequently do they occur, and whether other members of your family have migraine?

Better: At what age did your headaches start? (Answer)
  How often do they occur? (Answer)
  Do others in your family have migraine? (Answer)

False reassurance that makes unrealistic predictions or ignores the reality of the situation is not helpful.

The surgery will solve the problem. Don't worry about a thing.

I'm sure he still loves you.

The best reassurance is communicating by careful listening and examination that you understand the problem and have a positive plan of action.

Defensiveness is behavior on the part of the interviewer in response to feeling criticized by the patient.

I know other doctors might take an X-ray, but in *my* judgment it isn't necessary.

Just tell me your symptoms—I'll make the diagnosis.

If I thought you needed penicillin, I would have prescribed penicillin.

Vague Questions leave the patient unsure how to answer.

Do you lose your temper *often*?

Have you had this pain for *quite a while*?

Do you drink *very much* alcohol?

Has your general health been *good*?

The italicized words are so general that they are impossible to answer accurately. "Often" may mean once-a-day to one person and once every six months to another person. "Good health" means widely differing things to different people.

Vague statements are also too general to be interpreted properly.

Take it *easy* for a *few days*.

Relax. Don't worry. Don't let it upset you.

Do you have headaches or *anything like that*?

Forcing cooperation or compliance really leaves the patient no choice.

I want you to take this medication every three hours around the clock—OK?

This will hurt now—all right?

People are not diseases. People should not be referred to as "spastics," "epileptics," "hypertensives," "diabetics," "chronic lungers." There is a world of difference between asking "How long has Billy had epilepsy?" and "How long has Billy been an epileptic?" Words determine perceptions. Labeling people as diseases, a common practice among health care professionals, is a step towards dehumanizing patients (Moser, 1975).

Negative Phrasing

You don't have any heart trouble do you?

You haven't had any bleeding, have you?

No pain. (Meant as a question but put in the form of an assertion.)

Negative phrasing implies that you would not expect the patient to experience the item you are asking about. Some patients may not have the courage to correct you, but at the same time they are left wondering how important is the point in question. There is rarely a need for negative phrasing; any question to which you want just a Yes or No answer can be phrased in a neutral manner. The briefest way to ask such questions is by simply naming the subject with a questioning voice: "Heart trouble?" "Bleeding?" "Pain?"

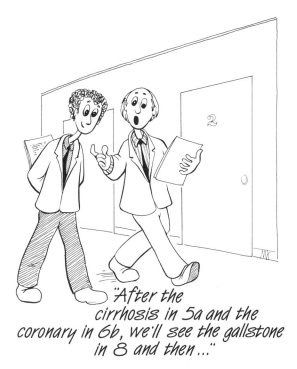

"After the cirrhosis in 5a and the coronary in 6b, we'll see the gallstone in 8 and then..."

People are not diseases.

This style is the only one that will get you through the Review of Systems in a reasonable time.

Jargon should be avoided. Don't use big words where little ones will do: "palpating" is feeling, "prognosis" is outlook, "therapy" is treatment. Anatomical terms, even the simplest, are a mystery to many persons, including well-educated ones. Medicine is filled with ponderous terms—avoid them with patients and colleagues. Also, address an adult in adult terms. To ask a grown person about "tummy pain" has a condescending quality. Some judgment is needed to match the education level of your patient to avoid being too technical or too simple; the key is to be aware of a tendency to use jargon. Tape recording your interviews is an ideal means of detecting the habit if you have developed it.

Apologetic questions

Could you tell me a *little bit* about why you are in the hospital?

Do you mind telling me why you have come to the hospital?

Introducing your questions in this way seems to say, "I'm just a medical student. I'm unsure of myself and I don't want you to get angry or impatient

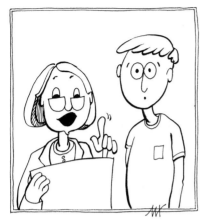

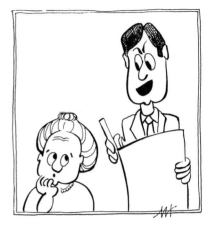

"I'D LIKE TO AUSCULTATE FOR MITRAL
INSUFFICIENCY"

"WHY DID YOU WAIT SO LONG TO
SEE A DOCTOR?"

Don't use big words where
little ones will do.

Avoid overtones of
accusation.

with me, so I am going to be as brief and untroubling as I can be." As discussed in *Chapter 2: Student Roles and Attitudes*, you have nothing to apologize for, and you should avoid communicating an attitude that diminishes your value or does not accurately reflect what you will be doing. A direct question helps establish the fact that you are in command of the situation.

☐ Information and Communication Theory

Communication is the foundation of the interview, as it is of social life generally. Information and communication theory are the "basic sciences" of interviewing, and will help you better understand and apply interviewing concepts. Several good books and articles on information and communication theory are listed in the *References and Readings* section at the end of this chapter.

Communication literally means "sharing"; when interviewing you share the thoughts, feelings, and behaviors associated with the patient's illness. Later, the patient shares your interpretation of the illness in terms of diagnosis, treatment plan, predictions about what to expect and general support. To achieve this sharing, the sender and receiver have a common language, or communication code, sent over some kind of communication channel (sight, hearing and sometimes touch in person-to-person communication).

The concept of communication as sharing of information differs from the general understanding of communication as a sending of new information the receiver does not previously have. In fact, the receiver must have all the elements of the information your message contains, otherwise communication is not possible. Given a range of possible meanings, communication is essentially a process of reducing uncertainty about which of the possible meanings is the one intended.

If the sender is Chinese and the receiver is English, the meaning imbedded in the Chinese language will not be accessible to the English listener at the verbal level. A separate channel of communication exists, however, that substitutes for or modifies verbal communication. *Nonverbal communication* has some universally understood elements. If the Chinese person smiles and extends his hand, for example, the English person is reasonably safe in assuming that a message of friendship is intended.

Verbal and nonverbal communication take place within an environment that reduces the possibility of error created by "noise" in the communication channel. Language is highly *redundant*; that is, within words and sentences are built-in duplications and accuracy checks that reduce the chance of error. For example, if A is talking to B on a very noisy telephone circuit, B might hear something like, "I'm bringing home a stone for the dog." How B interprets the message is a function of the context and of parallel knowledge—whether the couple has a pet frog or a dog at home, for example. When a physician asks, "How are you?" the meaning of the question is partly a function of where the question is asked. If spoken in the physician's office to a person who made an appointment because of an illness, the question is a request for health-related information. If the same two persons meet casually on the street, the question will be understood to be a form of social greeting.

In addition to context, redundancy is a property of language itself. It is possible to eliminate half the words from a newspaper article and still understand the essential report. If pictures or graphic displays accompany the article, an even greater percentage of the words can be eliminated without limiting the information content.

□ Communication Model

A model of communication is shown in the illustration.

The communication channel opens when you and your patient meet for a common health-related activity. Introducing yourself and identifying your role initiate the communication process. Active listening, acknowledgment, feedback, and other evidence of interest on your part keep the channel open. Similarly, the patient must be motivated to seek health care and must maintain confidence in you to keep the channel open. Jargon or unfamiliar terms distort the encoding/decoding process. Noise may take the form of interruption or distractions like telephone calls. Verbal and nonverbal messages, and their interrelations, are discussed in the next chapter.

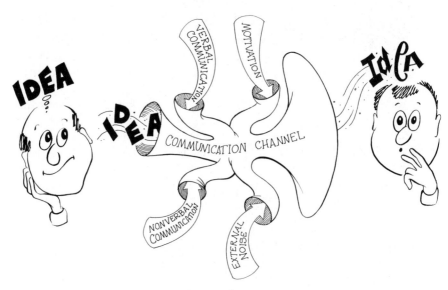

Model of Communication

☐ **REFERENCES AND READINGS**

Blois MS: Information and Medicine. Berkeley, University of California Press, 1984.
Campbell J: Grammatical Man. Information, Entropy, Language, and Life. New York, Simon and Schuster, 1982.
Cherry C: On Human Communication, ed 3. Cambridge, MA, MIT Press, 1978.
Information. Scientific American, September, 1966, entire issue.
Moser PH: People are not diseases (editorial). JAMA 1975; 233:62.
Morgan WL, Engel GL: The Clinical Approach to the Patient. Philadelphia, WB Saunders Co, 1969.
Northouse PG, Northouse LL: Health Communications: A Handbook for Health Professionals. Englewood Cliffs, NJ, Prentice-Hall, 1985.
Pierce JR: Symbols, Signals, and Noise. New York, Harper & Row, 1961.
Ruesch J: Communication and psychiatry. In Kaplan HI, Freedman AM, Sadock BJ (eds): Comprehensive Textbook of Psychiatry, ed 3. Baltimore, Williams & Wilkins, 1980, Chapter 4.7.
Swisher SN, Enelow AJ: Interviewing and Patient Care, ed 2. New York, Oxford University Press, 1979.
Watzlawick P, Beavin JH, Jackson DD: Pragmatics of Human Communication. New York, WW Norton, 1967.

CHAPTER 15

NONVERBAL COMMUNICATION

Daniel Levinson, MD
Robert E Rakel, MD*

Intended and Unintended
  Communication
Rapport and Nonverbal
  Communication
Classifying Nonverbal
  Communication
Kinesics (Body Language)
Touch
Paralanguage
Proxemics (Territoriality)
Artifacts
Physical Environment
Culture
Putting It All Together

Thus far we have focused on the verbal, or spoken interaction between you and your patient—the questions, answers, and expressions that establish the relationship, initiate the diagnostic process, and assist therapy. But as you and the patient talk, each of you also communicates on another level, the nonverbal, which is as significant in information transfer as is spoken communication.

☐ Intended and Unintended Communication

To better appreciate the power of nonverbal communication in the clinical setting, you need to recognize the distinction between *intended* and *unintended* communication. Intended communication transfers information you want the other person to have; unintended messages transfer information that you either are unaware of giving, or may wish not to reveal. Goffman (1959) refers to "information given" and "information given off." For example, a person wishes to create an impression of success by wearing an expensive-appearing watch. You, however, recognize the watch as a cheap imitation of an expensive brand. The patient says he drinks alcohol only on rare social occasions, but you note the odor of alcohol on his breath. The deliberate purchase of an expensive-appearing watch, and the statement about how often he drinks alcohol are intended communications; the small details of the watch that mark it as an

---

*Professor and Chairman, Department of Family Medicine, and Associate Dean for Academic and Clinical Affairs, Baylor College of Medicine, Houston, Texas.

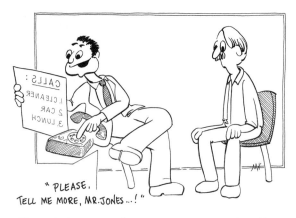

"PLEASE, TELL ME MORE, MR. JONES...!"

Nonverbal communication may contradict the verbal message.

imitation and the odor of alcohol are unintended communications. You may make other observations of which the patient is unaware that communicate the true state of affairs: a tremor, a soiled necktie, bruises suggesting a recent fall. Similarly, personal maturity, happiness, and a feeling of success are reflected nonverbally in many small ways.

Much of nonverbal communication deals with unintended messages. The distinction between intended and unintended messages touches on deception; in fact, some attorneys hire a communication specialist to be in court to search for signs that a witness may be lying. Cues to a hidden agenda, often the real reason for a patient seeking help, are usually nonverbal. But beyond deception or hidden agendas, we are always observing others, and they us, for all kinds of information about which neither person is aware. Verbal and nonverbal communication cannot be separated; they are both essential components of any interview.

When you perceive a contradiction between intended and unintended communication, the nonverbal information is usually a more accurate expression of thoughts and feelings than consciously controlled speech. For example, a hospitalized patient, when asked, "How are you today?" says, "Fine," but the patient's facial expression, quality of voice, and posture may all suggest a mood of depression. Other nonverbal messages, taken in at a glance, confirm the impression of depression: neglect of personal appearance, slight tearing, barely touched food, unopened mail on the bedside table, a mound of damp facial tissues. Also, you often know when a patient is doing well the minute you walk into the room; there is a sense of strength and optimism reflected in the patient's appearance and manner.

☐ Rapport and Nonverbal Communication

"Active listening," an important element of rapport, involves your perception of both the verbal and nonverbal messages the patient is sending. Most people "put on a front"—playing social roles that portray themselves as they would like to be regarded by others. Beneath role behavior, however, are feelings of vulnerability, shame or guilt, loneliness and other attitudes and emotions that the patient would benefit from sharing, if the sharing could be done safely. The ability to see beyond the surface, and to communicate both your understanding and acceptance of the *real* person behind the mask, creates a powerful bond of trust. Your sensitivity to messages "given off," rather than what the patient tells you with words, is often the key establishing a helping relationship.

Spoken communication in the clinical setting tends to deal with facts. Feelings, emotions, and values are less often communicated verbally. Nonverbal behavior is the basic medium by which feelings and emotions are communicated. Your ability to recognize and respond to these cues to patients' feelings and emotions is as important in establishing rapport as is your ability to understand the facts of a patient's illness. As with other areas of human functioning in which a person feels vulnerable, you must take the initiative if disturbances in the affective realm are to be recognized and openly discussed.

Just as you monitor a patient's nonverbal behavior, so do patients monitor yours. You will give off unintended communication to patients. A frown or a "Hmmm" of uncertainty may be misinterpreted as evidence that something serious is the matter. Nor will you be able to keep bad news from the patient.

A 70-year-old woman was admitted for evaluation of abdominal pain and marked weight loss. Noninvasive diagnostic studies were inconclusive, and an exploratory laparotomy was performed. Inoperable cancer was present. No one told her what was found at surgery, but she correctly guessed because her regular physician, who had visited her daily in the pre-operative period, stopped visiting her after the operation.

A patient who is lied to, even by omission, usually has available plenty of nonverbal information containing the truth, and will distrust family, friends, and physician if they persist in the charade.

□ Classifying Nonverbal Communication

Nonverbal communication has been classified in seven categories by Knapp (1978):

Kinesics: (Body Language). Gestures, posture, facial expression, eye appearance, gait. Examples include a forced smile, slight tearing, pounding the table.

Physical characteristics: Evidence of state of health, body shape, skin color, hair, deformities, characteristic body odors (diabetes, uremia, alcohol).

Touching: Handshake, hitting, skill with which physical examination is done.

Paralanguage: Voice pitch, inflection, rhythm, tempo, groaning, and expressions such as "uh huh," "ah," "well," "you know."

Proxemics: Personal space, seating arrangements at meetings, distance between individuals while in conversation.

Artifacts: Clothing, make-up, eyeglasses, jewelry. For example, excessive make-up is suggestive of a hysterical personality; wearing expensive clothes gives the impression of wealth.

Environment: Temperature, architecture, background sound, furniture, room decorations, contents of a hospital bedside table (a bedside stand devoid of cards, letters, or flowers, or filled with notes and flowers).

☐ Kinesics (Body Language)

Gestures or other body movements are rich in meaning. By themselves, or accompanying speech, they

1. *Substitute for speech*, as when pointing out a location of a symptom, or pointing a thumb down to indicate disapproval. Signing, a form of communication for deaf persons, is an entire language of gestures.

2. *Emphasize* a spoken communication. Pounding on a table, or striking a palm with a fist, indicates that the speaker feels strongly about the point being discussed.

3. *Illustrate.* You may find it easier to hold your cupped hands apart to indicate the size of a huge ovarian cyst just removed at surgery than to describe it with words.

4. *Show feelings.* The smile, for example, is a universal expression of pleasure and acceptance.

5. *Regulate speech.* Placing your palm up or touching your finger to your lips, both communicate, "Not so loud."

6. *Act as self-adaptors.* Gestures like clearing the throat, holding the head, straightening a necktie, or smoothing a dress seem to aid in reducing temporary stress.

These gestures may contain either intended or unintended information. The smile, for example, is often just what it appears to be—a spontaneous, honest reflection of pleasure. But smiles are also deliberately turned on at will, as beauty queen contestants learn to do as they go on stage before the judges. Professional actors master a wide repertoire of gestures. Patients often force a smile as a form of denial of concern.

Body Position. Posture reflects varying degrees of tension or relaxation. The tense person, for example, sits erect with a fairly rigid posture, while a relaxed person leans forward and sideways. An erect posture conveys an image of confidence and competence. Energetic people seldom slump; they sit upright and appear alert.

When rapport exists between two people, each mirrors the other's movements. Disruptions in this mirroring process signal that one member disagrees with what the other has said or feels betrayed or insulted but cannot express this verbally. Renegotiation or further explanation is indicated. *Depression* is reflected in posture and body movements.

A seriously depressed patient on the psychiatry service constantly asked the time. His wrist watch—a self-winding type—had stopped. The reason the watch stopped was evident in watching him walk. In the depths of his depression his arms hung limply at his sides as he shuffled along. There wasn't enough arm movement to wind the watch. As his depression lifted and his arms swung normally again, he no longer had to ask the time.

Face. Basic facial expressions of emotion are independent of culture. Joy, sadness, and anger are the same in the Australian aborigine, the American farmer, and the Norwegian fisherman. It is possible to control or disguise the facial expression, however. In the American culture, the mouth is most commonly used to conceal feelings. A person in a social gathering may be smiling, although inwardly sad or angry. The eyebrows, eyes, and forehead are least affected by learned disguises and are the most consistently dependable indicators of emotion. As Shakespeare wrote, "I saw his heart in his face" (The Winter's Tale, Act I, Scene II).

Head Position. Typically, the head is held forward in anger, back in defiance, anxiety, or fear, and down or bowed in sadness, submissiveness, shame, or guilt. When listening to a patient, your interest and concern is demonstrated by an attentive position—sitting forward in the chair with an attentive expression and the head slightly tilted.

Eyes. The eyes are a major organ of expression. They are so important to a person's appearance that when anonymity is desired, only the eyes need be covered. Surprise, anger, sincerity, fear, depression and other emotions can be read in a person's eyes, although the exact cues are difficult to describe. Sadness, while sometimes causing overt tears, is often reflected in a slight glistening of moisture where the lower lid meets the eye. Happiness, too, shows up in the eyes as a lively sparkle.

Eye Contact. Eye contact accompanies a special kind of human-to-human awareness. Frequent eye contact conveys interest. A listener who does not maintain eye contact, but looks down or away from the speaker may be shy, lack self-esteem, be depressed, or is expressing resistance to the speaker or the comments being made. Prolonged gaze, or staring, in most cultures is unpleasant, but failing to exchange glances can be dehumanizing and cause the patient to feel more like an object than a person.

The frequency of eye contact provides clues about a person's mood. Depressed patients, for example, maintain eye contact only one fourth of the time of nondepressed patients. Anxious patients may maintain eye contact more than usual or may move their eyes more frequently from the physician to other objects in the room.

Hands. The hands droop with sadness, and are clenched when responding to anger. The "white knuckles" of tightly locked fingers are often a sign of anxiety, which may also be expressed by tremor. Joining hands, with fingers extended and fingertips touching, called *steepling*, indicates confidence and assurance in the comments being made.

A slight raising of the hand, or perhaps only the index finger, is a subtle indicator of the urge to interrupt, indicating that the patient wants to share important information. A patient listening in "The Thinker" position, but with the index finger extended along the cheek, or sitting with elbows on the table and hands clenched in front of the mouth while listening intently may not be buying what the physician is saying, indicating a need to check out acceptance with the patient.

Arms. Folded arms, a gesture found in all cultures, is a natural position of comfort; however, it also communicates learned messages of defensiveness, disagreement, or insecurity. If the posture suggests resistance or defensiveness, search for the reason. Perhaps a recommendation to stop smoking, for example, is threatening and difficult to accept. If so, you will need to make an additional effort to explain the rationale for the recommendation.

Legs. Although crossing the legs is a common position of comfort, it also indicates a shutting out of, or protection against, the outside world. If crossed legs confirm the total kinesic picture of resistance including crossed arms, make an effort to identify the reason for the resistance. A resistant patient is likely to provide incomplete information and reject your therapeutic recommendations. Note the position and movement of feet. Just as anxiety is associated with fidgety hand movements, it is also indicated by constantly moving feet. An anxious or scared person may sit forward in the chair with feet placed in the "ready to run" position, one foot in front of the other. Widely spaced feet may indicate anger, whereas a sad person's feet move in a slow, circular pattern.

☐ Touch

Touch communicates a close personal interest in the patient, and often is an important part of establishing rapport, as discussed in *Chapter 4: Rapport.* In the United States the handshake is the most socially acceptable method of touch, and indicates the wish for a positive relationship. The handshake as a traditional greeting of friendship began with the custom of raising exposed hands as evidence that no weapons were held. A limp handshake communicates insecurity or fear. A moist palm is a sign of nervousness or apprehension, and the "halfway-there," fingers-only handshake reflects reluctance or indecision.

Other forms of touch that communicate your concern, support, and reassurance include stroking and holding. Stroking, a special kind of touching, may be no more than a fleeting touch on the forearm or shoulder. Holding, sometimes needed to calm a frightened or uncontrolled child or adult, done in a firm but considerate manner, helps the patient regain confidence and self-control. During labor women instinctively reach out to the attending doctor, nurse, or spouse to hold hands when labor pains climax.

Although touch is valuable in a clinical interaction, its use is not mandatory. Each of you has your own ways of expressing interest in others. If touch is not comfortable for you, its use would be artificial and insincere. Furthermore, some patients do not like to be touched, and may misinterpret such behaviors as seductive.

□ Paralanguage

Paralanguage is the voice *qualities* that accompany or modify speech. Velocity of speech (fast, flow, hesitant), tone, volume, sighs and grunts, pauses, and inflections have meanings not contained in words as such. Consider the differences in meaning of the same sentence spoken with differing emphasis:

- □ "Is *that* all that bothers you?" A trivial problem, not worth the concern being giving it.
- □ "Is that *all* that bothers you?" Is there something else troubling the patient?
- □ "Is that all that *bothers* you?" I only want to hear about significant problems, not everything that might be a problem

A rapid-fire, clipped speaking pattern is characteristic of the "Type A" personality thought by some as a marker of risk of myocardial infarction. Urgency, sincerity, confidence, hesitation, thoughtfulness, gaiety, sadness, and apprehension are all conveyed by qualities of voice. Subtle changes of tone signal unspoken fear, doubts, or the unspoken need for reassurance. Frequent pauses and "ahh's" communicate uncertainty or perhaps attempted deception. The frequent, sometimes annoying, clearing of the voice (the respiratory avoidance response [RAR]), suggests rejection or disgust, either by the patient or the physician. *Forced* laughter, rather than communicating humor, often signals the presence of unpleasant thoughts and feelings.

Tone of voice can actually reverse the meaning of words; when the verbal and nonverbal messages transmit contradictory information, the nonverbal is usually the more accurate. Sarcasm is a common example of the contradiction between spoken and nonverbal messages. Paralanguage is particularly helpful in interpreting telephone conversations. For example, a patient with a history of recurring depression answered the phone with an up-rising "Hello" when feeling well, but with a downward "Hello" when feeling depressed. The urgency of a telephone request is reflected as much in the quality of the caller's voice as in the verbal message.

☐ Proxemics (Territoriality)

Territoriality, a fundamental fact of animal life, has its counterpart in human behavior. Standing too close to another person creates tension and uneasiness unless there is a mutual desire for intimacy. On the other hand, too much space between persons discourages serious conversation. In addition, barriers such as a table communicate "Keep your distance." When setting up your office you will want to give some thought to where you will situate your desk in relation to the patient, since seating arrangements offer you a chance to control the degree of psychological closeness you feel is right for you. Many physicians find placement of the patient's chair at the side of the desk encourages better communication than if physician and patient talk to each other across a table. In some offices the interview is conducted with facing chairs only.

Your spatial relationship to a patient in a bed also influences the doctor-patient relationship. Standing while talking with a patient communicates your intent to stay only a few minutes—not enough time for substantiative communication—and reinforces the passive role of patients inherent in much of health care. Sitting, rather than standing, communicates that you plan to spend some time with the patient and equalizes the interpersonal relationship. In caring for young children, you will want to think about how a child might feel looking up at a large adult. Usually you can find a less threatening position from which to talk and examine the child.

☐ Artifacts

Clothing, make-up, eyeglasses, jewelry, in fact everyting patients select to wear or apply to their body reflects the persons' self-regarding attitude and the kind of impression they wish to create in others.

When a woman, recovering from a serious illness or operation, starts using make-up again, you can be sure the recuperation is going well. Women with a histrionic, hysterical personality characteristically wear bold, excessive make-up and prefer sexually seductive clothes. Such women usually exaggerate their descriptions of illness, and are subject to conversion reactions that mimic disease with astonishing fidelity. (This does not mean that hysterical persons never get organic disease—only that interpreting their symptoms is a complex challenge.)

□ Physical Environment

Physical surroundings communicate a lot about the person occupying an area. Surroundings also facilitate or inhibit communication. Interviewing requires a quiet, private area. The presence of other persons, constant interruption, or distracting noise from a radio or television set, impose limits on an interview. Other physical factors influencing the interview include furniture, air temperature and humidity, lighting, and room dividers. A simple bedside hospital table tells a great deal about the patient.

Elderly Mrs. Jacobs was demanding and critical of everything in the hospital. She had no use for anyone on the staff, with one exception—Paul, the fourth-year medical student. She would do anything Paul asked, and do it cheerfully. We couldn't understand Paul's magic until one day we noted a picture on Mrs. Jacobs' bedside table of a young man who bore a striking resemblance to Paul. It was a picture of her only grandson, whom she worshipped. The bedside table explained all.

In addition to influencing the interview, surroundings communicate important information. A physician's office, tastefully decorated, with recent magazines and comfortable chairs in the reception area, reflects concern for patients' comfort. Similarly, home surroundings provide an understanding of a patient that office or hospital contacts cannot possibly communicate. No other activity can tell you as much about a patient's life in a brief time as does a house call.

□ Culture

Interpreting a nonverbal observation isolated from the total context is risky. In general, verbal and nonverbal communication constitute a unit; each is understood in the context of the other. While some nonverbal behaviors, such as smiling and laughter, are universal in meaning, many other behaviors are learned in the process of growing up within a particular culture. Cultural differences may assign altogether different meanings to the same behavior (the American "A-OK" gesture is an obscene sign in some foreign countries).

The nature of a person's eye contact says a lot about the person's culture. In the United States, focusing one's eyes on the speaker indicates respect and attention regardless of the age of the individuals involved. However, Hispanics and Blacks tend not to maintain as much eye contact while listening as do other Americans, and may look away from the speaker more often. This is not a sign of disrespect or inattention. In Latin American countries, a younger person is thought disrespectful if his eyes meet those of the adult who is speaking. A physician who maintained steady eye contact while talking to a patient would risk being considered seductive in that culture. Looking away from the speaker from time to time may be a sign of respect and sensitivity rather than the opposite. What is true of eye contact in terms of cultural influence is true of most other kinds of nonverbal behavior. Obviously, the physician needs to consider the patient's cultural background when interpreting the meaning of nonverbal behavior.

□ Putting It All Together

Analyzing nonverbal communication in a textbook artificially dissects what in reality is a blend of behaviors. The intuitive, unconscious processing of intended and unintended clues is suggested by the following example:

One Saturday evening a young man, about 25, walked up to the emergency room rather slowly and asked to see a doctor because of "stomach pain." The doctor was at the reception desk and saw the patient walk in; immediately he thought "appendicitis," a diagnosis that proved to be correct.

How did a brief glance correctly identify the problem? Nonverbal information (a slow gait, a slight forward bend of the body, perhaps a strained facial expression), the awareness that most young men don't come to an emergency room on a Saturday night unless really sick, plus the knowledge that the most common significant abdominal condition in this age group is appendicitis all entered into the intuitive diagosis.

These are not the criteria for diagnosing appendicitis found in standard textbooks. Intuition is not in itself a recommended basis for performing surgery, but informed intuition, based on repeated observations, generates diagnostic considerations that may be as accurate as conventional symptoms, signs, and laboratory test results. The more direct clinical contact with patients you have (even if you don't understand everything you see), the more reliable will be your intuition.

□ Conclusion

Alan Alda (1979), in a medical school commencement address, challenged new physicians to read a patient's nonverbal messages as well as they read patients' x-rays. He said:

Can you see the fear and uncertainty in my face? If I tell you where it hurts, can you hear in my voice where I ache? I show you my body but I bring you my person. Will you tell me what you are doing and in words I can understand? Will you tell me when you don't know what to do? You will see the fear and uncertainty in the patient's face only if you look at the patient rather than at the medical record.

Alda's statement reflects the concern and compassion that patients desire and which your nonverbal messages will convey in a manner not possible by words alone.

□ REFERENCES AND READINGS

This chapter does no more than outline the importance of nonverbal communication in every phase of social interaction. If you want to look further into the subject, the following will be useful.

Alda A: Time Magazine May 28, 1979, p 68.
Blanch PD, Buck R, Rosenthal R: Nonverbal Communications in the Clinical Context. University Park, PA, Pennsylvania State University Press, 1986.
Goffman E: The Presentation of Self in Everyday Life. New York, Doubleday, 1959.
Knapp ML: Nonverbal Communication in Human Interaction. New York, Holt, Rinehart and Winston, 1978.
Rakel RE, Levinson D: Establishing Rapport. In Rakel RE (ed): Textbook of Family Practice, ed 3. Philadelphia, WB Saunders Company, 1984, Chapter 26.

UNIT V

INTERVIEW PROCEDURES

CHAPTER 16

PROCEDURE BASICS

Having considered the theory of interviewing, it is time to look at the practical, how-to-do-it aspects. This chapter focuses primarily on the interview process; you may want to review *Chapter 9: The Problem-Centered Interview* and *Chapter 12: The Health Promotion Interview* for interview content, which is not detailed here.

☐ Creating a Relationship

☐ THE INTERVIEWER: NAME AND ROLE

As soon as you meet your assigned patient, identify yourself by name and role. Patients frequently get confused by the number of health care professionals. Writing out your name is a thoughtful courtesy. Your role as a medical student should be explained. Be sure you wear a name tag (although some are so small that only people with excellent eyesight are able to read it). Don't apologize for your student status; you often have an important part to play as a member of the health care team. (You may find it helpful to review *Chapter 2: Student Roles and Concerns.*)

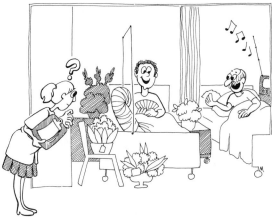

Evaluate the physical setting of the interview.

□ THE PATIENT

Have you correctly identified the patient? Did you pronounce the name correctly? Be sure you have the assigned patient; every so often, in the rush of care on the unit, the wrong patient is taken to surgery or given treatment intended for someone else.

In recent years, calling adult patients by their first names, even on the patient's first visit, has become fashionable. The intent is to put the patient at ease and to diminish the authoritarian stance associated with the medical profession. A "Hello, Millie, I am Dr. Jones" actually emphasizes differences. Furthermore, a first name relationship carries with it a sense of personal familiarity that restricts your options and ability to set limits or deal with truths the patient may prefer to avoid. Rapport and professionalism do not depend on familiarity. If you feel this is an issue, you can ask what the patient would like to be called, but do so in a way that doesn't impose your wishes. The safest course is to start off with "Mr." or "Mrs." or "Ms." and see where the relationship goes over time and repeated contact. Gradually going from a more formal to a less formal relationship over time is a natural evolution; the reverse is awkward, perhaps impossible without straining the relationship. With children and teenagers, a first-name relationship is natural and appropriate.

□ COMFORT

Inquire about the patient's comfort, and do whatever you can to put the patient at ease. An interview may last an hour or more—arrange things so that the patient doesn't have to assume an awkward position to talk with you.

You should be comfortable, too. Find a suitable chair and arrange it so that you and the patient can interact easily. If you are not relaxed, patients will sense your situation and limit what they tell you. Avoid starting an interview when you are upset or distracted by personal problems; patients can usually tell your distress and may mistakenly believe you have adverse information about their condition.

□ THE SETTING

Evaluate the physical setting of the interview. Is privacy assured? If not, your patient will not speak freely. A curtain does not provide complete privacy, as others in the room may be able to overhear. Is the room free from noise and distractions such as a television set? Don't be shy about asking that the set be turned off while you are with the patient. Are there time or schedule conflicts—is the patient expecting visitors, for example? If so, could you do your interview at a different time? If not, give the visitor an estimate of when you will be finished. Diagnostic and treatment procedures, of course, take priority over your assignment.

□ EQUIPMENT

Are you equipped with note paper, writing instruments, and a check list to guide the interview? Nothing else is necessary, although a box of facial tissues near at hand is appreciated if a patient cries when dealing with emotional issues. Simply handing the patient the box of tissues communicates that you understand and accept these feelings. (Having nothing better to offer a crying patient than the sleeve of your white coat is a bit awkward.)

□ Language, Cultural Background, and Motivation

You'll want to be sure significant language problems won't interfere with the interview. Many hospitals have staff persons who speak a language in addition to English, or an interpreter on-call who can help you with communication. Some hospitals have a Translator Bank—persons in the community who can be called on short notice to provide translations. Interpreters introduce complications into the health care process, however. Problems include lack of equivalent medical terms in different languages, nonverbal gestures with culturally different meanings, different health belief systems, and time and cost constraints in a busy clinic. The presence of the interpreter in the examination room creates problems of confidentiality, embarrassment when discussing personal information or disrobing, and emotional involvement if the translator is a friend or family member (Putsch, 1985; Faust and Dricky, 1986). Nothing is as satisfactory as speaking a foreign language yourself. Some medical schools offer elective courses in Spanish, and perhaps other languages.

If your patient is deaf, a person able to use sign language can act as an interpreter, or you can use a questionnaire.

Other early assessments include learning about motivation—did the patient come voluntarily, because of family insistence, or other external pressures? Identifying the patient's cultural background will help you know how to interpret culturally determined behaviors. Patients from Mediterranean countries, for example, may dramatize their symptoms with emotional displays, whereas persons from Far Eastern cultures often remain stoic or even smile in the face of discomfort. These issues have been discussed in *Chapter 3: Seeking and Accepting Health Care.*

□ Mental Status and Patient Reliability

Within a few minutes after meeting your patient, make an assessment of the patient's *reliability.* Persons who are in severe pain, heavily sedated, depressed, or suffering from acute or chronic brain impairment are unable to supply you with an accurate history. Such conditions affect memory, attention, and other intellectual abilities upon which accurate information depends. Patients may hide their intellectual impairment by evasion, fabricating stories, being overly pleasant or being unexpectedly hostile. In these circumstances, information from other sources such as relatives and prior records is necessary.

If you question the patient's reliability based on mental or central nervous system impairment, perform a simple *mental status examination.* The following is a brief screening format:

Recent memory: What did you have for breakfast?

Remote memory: Where were you born?

Orientation: What is today's date? Where are you right now?

Attention and Concentration: Count backwards from 20.

General Knowledge: Who is the president?

For a detailed discussion of the mental status examination and its correlation with disease processes, see Strub and Black, 1977, or standard psychiatry or neurology textbooks. Pfeiffer, 1975, has devised a short questionnaire that can be scored.

Gently introduced ("Mr. Jones, you seem to be having some memory trouble. I am going to ask you a few memory questions."), this examination will be enough to evaluate reliability. A complete mental status examination is usually part of the neurological examination or a special psychiatric evaluation, but a brief assessment takes only a few minutes and is essential at the onset of any interview if the patient's behavior, appearance, or response to initial questions suggests cognitive impairment.

Evidence of cognitive impairment does not mean there is no value in talking further with the patient. You will not be able to rely on the facts the patient relates, but the *form* of error or distortion is often of diagnostic value. A statement or implication that previous doctors prescribed "poison" suggests paranoia; inaccuracy in recall of recent, but not past, events is consistent with organic brain impairment; a rambling, hard-to-follow story, with sudden changes from one topic to the next, often is evidence of schizophrenia as in the following statement, spoken in a monotone, from a 16-year-old who had come to an arthritis clinic because

...my joints seem to have little snapping noises, and when I move my leg or something I hear a little snap, like a snap, (pause) ... just like the bones were rubbing against ... no, not like that, (pause) ... like in a certain position they would stay like they would be in that position, and then when I move to another position in order to, instead of moving along with the motion, it goes from that motion to it...and it doesn't follow through with the main idea of motion in that direction, you know ...

The fact that a patient is factually unreliable does not mean that there is no chance of using the interview to establish a relationship. Actually, such persons are often aware of their shortcomings, are exquisitely sensitive to their caretakers' attitudes, and are capable of developing close and meaningful ties.

Reliability of information obtained during the interview is also determined by what the patient can be reasonably expected to know about past events. The more distant an event, the less likely is a person to have accurate recall. When patients with peptic ulcers were asked the details of a previous hospital admission, significant discrepancies were found between what the patient said during the interview and the facts that were in the record of the past admission (Corwin et al, 1971). Neugent and Neugent (1984) found an error rate as high as 47 percent in the information about past illnesses provided during interviews in an emergency room setting. Also, many persons have never known the facts to begin with. This is especially true with the Family Medical History (Hastrup et al, 1985). In cases in which certain facts are essential and the patient's recall is uncertain, information must be obtained from other sources such as old records or informed relatives.

□ The Broad Picture

Initiate the questioning phase of the interview with a general query such as "How can I be of help?" "Why have you come to the hospital (or clinic)?"

or "What kind of problem are you having?" Then get an unstructured overview, from the patient's point of view, of the current problem, its setting, course, and importance to the patient. An open-ended, "Tell me more about it" style is best. This information helps you decide on the subsequent course of the interview, avoiding false starts and missing the patient's true concern.

Open-ended or unstructured questioning, discussed in detail in *Chapter 14: Verbal (Spoken) Techniques*, is both a valuable questioning technique, and even more importantly, an attitude. Frequently the interviewer structures the entire interview according to the initial, and sometimes incorrect, impression of what is wrong with the patient. Such preconceptions fundamentally alter the truth of the situation.

☐ Present Illness

☐ CAUSAL OR RISK FACTORS

- ☐ Past Health History.
- ☐ Family Health History (Hereditary/Contagious History).
- ☐ Personal/Social History (Life Style).

A Health Promotion interview will be much more detailed than a Problem-Centered interview. Instead of a limited, selective Review of Systems, for example, you do a complete ROS. Similarly, you should obtain a complete Personal/Social History that provides a comprehensive "patient profile."

In every interview, however brief, ask yourself if you have considered these *Fundamental Four* areas of health-related information. In some situations one or more of these major categories can be omitted. Often, however, so much time is spent in getting the details of the Present Illness that not even a single open-ended question is asked about Past Medical History, Family Medical History, or Personal/Social History. *It is easy to return to any area of the medical history for more details after you have the overall picture in mind.* If, however, you focus entirely on a single aspect of the patient's problem, it is possible to overlook some important factor in the patient's overall situation. The process is like selecting a place to live: you first "look over the field" in terms of price, location, and number of rooms; only after making broad decisions do you look into details like dripping faucets and stuck windows.

☐ Closing the Interview

In some ways, the last few minutes of the interview may be the most productive. Summarizing the major points of the interview reminds the patient of important information to be added. Also, the patient has had a chance to get to know you and may decide you are "OK" and can be trusted with information not previously mentioned. Indicating you are about through may signal a last chance to express what is really the concern. Listen for a too casual, "Oh, by the way, I was just wondering if . . ." question as you are about to leave. This may disclose what really has been on the patient's mind all along. It is better to leave the patient after asking three final questions.

□ THREE FINAL QUESTIONS

1. Anything else to add?
"We've discussed many things. Is there anything at all that you would like to bring up or discuss further?"
2. Does the patient have questions?
"I've asked you a lot of questions. Perhaps there are questions you would like to ask me."
Often a patient needs only information to solve the problem. See *Chapter 19: The Interview as Therapy and Patient Education.*
3. What are the patient's ideas and concerns about the current problem?
"I'd be interested in knowing what you think is wrong" (or causing the problem, or similar phrases).
Sometimes unexpected ideas, misconceptions, or fears not expressed during the interview emerge:
"I'm really afraid it's cancer—just like my mother had when she was my age."
Often the patient has a very good idea of what is wrong:
"If you really want to know, I think it's all due to my job—I hate *every* minute of it!"
"I'm terribly worried about my children—I worry all the time. I think it's affecting my health."
Be sensitive to the extent to which the patient really wants a precise diagnosis. Often, all the patient is seeking is an answer to whether a symptom represents something serious. If reassured that the condition is not serious and will soon cure itself, many people are content to stop there and give the problem more time. They are satisfied with your just giving the condition a name or receiving a simple biological explanation. Misreading a request for information as a request for treatment converts a minor condition into one with the potential for complications. Starting an extensive evaluation entangles the patient in expense and inconvenience, and prescribing medications may cause side effects. Knowing when to reassure and when to pursue a full evaluation depends on experience, judgment, and willingness to tolerate a degree of uncertainty. This is why you have preceptors to guide you.
Other helpful methods of bringing the interview to a successful conclusion are:

□ Whenever appropriate, give a few "strokes." Let the patient know the information has been helpful and that you appreciate the time and effort invested. Many people see your interview as a privileged sort of personal test, and appreciate knowing they have "passed with flying colors."

☐ Whether or not to thank the patient depends on what your role has been. If it is evident that the interview was primarily for your educational benefit, the patient should indeed be thanked. If, on the other hand, you are a part of the clinical team, it is the patient who should thank you. In fact, thanks usually abound on both sides.

☐ Will you see the patient again? If so, let the patient know. Often a patient will keep a record of things to be brought up upon your return. If you will not see the patient again, the patient may want to express to you good wishes and perhaps other matters you will find helpful and pleasant.

☐ Too Much Information, or Too Little?

Most students get too much information, rather than too little. Does it really matter if a 45-year-old man had mumps when he was age 5, or age 10, or just that he had the disease? Having hard facts is reassuring—you feel like you are getting somewhere—but it is not always possible. If a patient obviously doesn't recall something, don't force an answer. Listen to yourself on tape; chances are you will hear yourself pushing the patient for an exact date or going over and over a detail that is unlikely to make much of a difference anyhow.

Finally, if you complete your interview in 10 minutes, that's fine. You may not believe your good luck, and you may keep going over the same things again and again. Some people have simple health histories that are easily obtained in a brief time—don't fight it.

☐ Interview Sequence

The interview sequence is not fixed. The *Fundamental Four* progression is flexible. If the patient's history logically takes some other sequence, or if you sense the patient wants to talk about a concern that you would otherwise come to later, that's fine as long as you complete all sections before finishing the interview. In some instances, information from one section of the history suggests that new information is available in some other section. For example, if you learn that the patient is taking medications commonly associated with heart disease and the patient has not mentioned a cardiac problem, you will want to review *Past Health History* again, asking specifically for what condition the heart medication is being taken. In addition, if you have not done a cardiovascular system review during the history of the Present Illness, doing so may produce useful new information about the patient's current health.

While flexibility in the interview allows the patient's history to develop in a natural order, following a routine is insurance against omission. A well-practiced routine becomes a habit—you follow it automatically, even at times of pressure when you might not have time for more deliberate interviewing. Also, the *Fundamental Four* framework helps you shift from one section to another in case you find yourself temporarily at a loss in any one line of questioning. "Hang loose" and you'll never be uncertain about what to do next.

□ Notetaking

Recording information as you obtain it from the patient is a constant problem for all clinicians. It is a particularly difficult challenge when the information doesn't form a meaningful pattern. Constantly writing notes during an interview distracts the patient and interferes with good communication. A useful notetaking technique is to obtain as much information as you can remember at one time, stop, summarize your understanding to the patient, and make a note. Then resume interviewing, summarize, and again write down what is essential. Don't be concerned about recording every detail of the past—get a broad overview. If you need more details, you can get them later. If you discover, as you write up the history, that you have forgotten something important (everyone does at times), or some new line of reasoning occurs to you after you have left the patient, go back for more interviewing when the time is appropriate. There is no law requiring perfect performance the first time, every time.

The interview and note-taking are just two aspects of a complex medical information system. In *Unit VII: Communication within the Profession* communication by spoken presentations and by written records is discussed. In *Unit VIII: Technical Supports* the use of checklists, forms that are designed to record information, questionnaires, and computers is reviewed.

□ Return Visits

Thus far we have described the interview of a patient who is entirely new to you and who has a new medical problem. After the initial visit or two, you should have recorded a complete database, and you will have most of the patient's history in mind. Return visits, therefore, are usually brief and focus on the Present Illness. You will want to know whether the initial symptoms are still present, changed for better or worse, or have disappeared as a result of therapy or the natural course of illness. Often developments open up new diagnostic possibilities; then you may have to reconsider the *Fundamental Four* for new information. Also, as the patient comes to know and trust you, facts may be confided for the first time. There is no better way to learn about the course of disease than observing patients over time. Visit your patients whenever possible, even if you are no longer on the service where your first contact was made.

☐ Reading

Immediately after seeing a patient is the ideal time to study that patient's disease. Optimal learning occurs in a context of relevance. Always have access to standard textbooks that describe the pathophysiological basis for disease as well as the distinguishing clinical findings. Compare the clinical picture of your patient to the textbook description (few real-life patients exactly match textbook descriptions). Reading may suggest new avenues to explore.

The patient's chart is a textbook of sorts, depending on the quality of entries made by members of the health care team. Often you will find interpretive discussions of the patient's disease. In any event, the record contains a wealth of clinical data upon which the diagnosis is based. (Look at the record *after* you have evaluated your patient; to read the clinical history and diagnosis of others before seeing the patient deprives you of a uniquely valuable experience of discovery and problem-solving.)

☐ REFERENCES AND READINGS

Beresford TP, Holt RE, Hall RC, et al: Cognitive screening at the bedside: Usefulness of a structured examination. Psychosomatics 1985; 26:319–324.

Corwin RG, Krober M, Roth HP: Patients' accuracy in reporting their past medical history. J Chron Dis 1971; 23:875–879.

Faust S, Dricky R: Working with interpreters. J Fam Pract 1986; 22:131–138.

Hastrup JL, Hotchkiss AP, Johnson CA: Accuracy of knowledge of family history of cardiovascular disorders. Health Psychology 1985; 4:291–306.

Neugent AI, Neugent RH: How accurate are patient histories? J Community Health 1984; 9:294–301.

Pfeiffer E: A short portable mental status questionnaire for reassessment of organ brain deficit in elderly patients. J Am Geriatr Soc 1975; 23:433–441.

Putsch RW: Cross-cultural communication: The special case of interpreters in health care. JAMA 1985; 254:3344–3348.

CHAPTER 17

INTERVIEWING IN THE HOSPITAL

☐ Preliminaries: The Hospital Unit

You are likely to begin your interviewing experience in a hospital rather than a doctor's office or outpatient setting. Knowing something about a hospital unit and how it operates will help you feel comfortable in what is sometimes an intimidating environment.

Each hospital unit is a small community administered by a *Head Nurse*, a Registered Nurse (RN) who has overall responsibility for everything that happens on the unit. Providing direct patient care are other RN *staff nurses, Licensed Practice Nurses* (LPN), and *Nurses' Aides* (NA). A *Unit Clerk* maintains charts, answers the telephone, welcomes visitors, locates supplies, and starts the physician's orders into motion.

☐ Physicians

Physicians usually are a part of *Clinical Services*, such as internal medicine, surgery, obstetrics/gynecology, or pediatrics, that care for patients in several units in the hospital. Heading a clinical service is the *Attending Physician*, who has ultimate responsibility for the medical care of the patient. The "attending" may also be the patient's personal physician, but in some hospitals, especially those that are a part of a university system, community physicians may not have appointments to the university hospital medical staff.

Serving with the Attending Physician are one or more *Residents*. The *First Year Resident* (also called an intern) has just graduated from medical school

159

and is not yet a licensed physician, since most states do not grant a license to practice until a Doctor of Medicine (an academic title, not a legal one) has had one year of experience of supervised practice as an intern or resident. Many clinical services have second, third, or fourth year residents, each having had added training and thus able to assume more responsibility. Finally, many hospitals have a *Chief Resident*, a person who has come up through the ranks of the residency and is now responsible for much of the day-to-day supervision of the resident staff. The Chief Resident is both an experienced clinician and an able administrator who knows how to get things done. The attending physician and the hospital staff depend heavily on this person's ability and judgment.

Fellows are often members of a hospital team. They are usually physicians, or sometimes PhD's, who spend part or most of their time in research, and who also have an interest in patient care.

Other members on the hospital staff you will want to know about, and meet if possible (don't be shy about asking), include:

□ Hospital Administrator.
□ Dietician or Nutritionist.
□ Medical Librarian.
□ Chaplain or Spiritual Advisor.
□ Chief Pharmacist.
□ Medical Records Administrator.

These people are only a few of the individuals who make a hospital function smoothly. Large hospitals have many other persons performing specialized services that ultimately affect patient care. A good way to quickly become acquainted with the organization of a hospital is to scan the Hospital Telephone Directory.

□ Rounds

The one occasion for everyone getting together is *Rounds* (Perrino et al, 1986). There may be several: *Teaching Rounds*, which emphasize the educational aspects of hospitalized patients, and *Work* or *Chart* Rounds, in which the focus is on the details of patient care.

□ When You Arrive On The Hospital Unit

When you are assigned to a patient on a hospital unit where you have not previously worked, the first thing to do is to introduce yourself to the Head Nurse (or whoever is in charge), and explain your assignment. Inquire about the patient you are to visit: Are there factors that might influence the interview? Can the bed position be changed? Is the patient medically stable and psychologically ready for your visit?

In many medical schools your preceptor will have discussed your visit with the patient ahead of time. If not, you'll have to do some negotiating on your own. There will be times when you will have to defer or even cancel the interview because of the needs of the patient and the unit.

Get to know how the unit operates and the responsibilities of each person there. Hospital personnel are usually very supportive of students and will help you in every way possible. Take the time to establish and maintain positive relationhips with them. Help out if you can—there are always opportunities. Don't be afraid to ask for help. Members of the team have a lot of valuable experience to share if you create the right kind of atmosphere. A friendly, helping relationship with the unit staff will ease many stressful times throughout your career.

□ Sequence of the Interview

The general order of the interview is the same as that described in *Chapter 16: Procedure Basics.* Some modification will be necessary, however, when your assigned patient has been in the hospital for some time—a frequent occurrence in teaching hospitals where the same patient may be interviewed several times. In this circumstance, the patient usually knows the diagnosis and is not a "new" patient in the sense of being admitted to the hospital at the onset of an illness. To gain the most value from interviewing such patients, you will have to modify your introductory questioning by saying something like

"I understand you have been in the hospital for some time now; however, for me to get a clear idea of your condition, could you go back to the beginning and tell me in what way you became ill?"

Sometimes the patient has been in the hospital so long, or for so many admissions as a result of complications or progression of a chronic condition, that the onset of the illness is no longer clear. In such instances, the Present Illness is the reason for the current hospitalization—an "illness within an illness." You will have to adapt your interview to the unique situation of each patient. Make each patient a challenge. Simply recording the events as the patient relates them, without trying to understand what they were like as they evolved, deprives you of a problem-solving opportunity.

□ After The Interview

After finishing the interview, or the interview and physical examination, be sure that the patient's bed is returned to its original position, especially if you have raised it. If you have used an examination room, cleaning up—throwing away gloves, replacing examination table paper, rinsing off instruments—is appreciated. Then let the Head Nurse know you are finished and the room is free to be used by others.

□ Staying in Contact With Your Patients

Even if you are just beginning your interview experience and are not a part of the ward team, you might want to follow a patient you have interviewed. A daily visit provides invaluable experience in learning about the course of illness. Also, repeated visits help you develop skills in maintaining a relationship. Many patients will welcome your visit and will sometimes share information, based on their experience as a patient, which you can learn in no other way. If you sense a meaningful interaction, encourage the relationship. It is important that you avoid making statements that might conflict with the patient's management, and that the attending physician know of your interest in visiting the patient.

□ Hospital Records

The hospital record is available to you; don't hesitate to consult it *after* you have seen the patient and completed your write-up. Looking at the record before doing your interview deprives you of a valuable learning opportunity. It is difficult to avoid being biased by a previous examiner's clinical impression.* Every new patient should be an opportunity for *discovery*, not merely confirmation. Don't overlook the possibility that the initial diagnosis in the chart is wrong or incomplete and that you may perceive the patient's problem in a fresh, more accurate way.

Remember when reading the chart that there is only one record—never, under any circumstances, remove it from the unit work area. With the paper-based record system used by most hospitals, only one person at a time has access to a patient's chart. The whole health care process comes to a halt while the staff searches for a missing chart. When records are computerizd, as they will be some day, patient care information will be available to every member of the staff when and where needed.

When looking through a chart, read the Nurses' Notes. The nurses observe the patient 24 hours a day, and their observations are invaluable in knowing

---

*Gross (1971) describes an epidemic disease found in teaching centers, which he calls "The Emperor's New Clothes Syndrome." This contagious condition starts when a senior member of the rounding team detects some minimal or nonexistent physical finding such as a faint heart murmur. No one else detects it, but "down the line, in rapid succession, members of the group are infected." Gross advises that to avoid becoming infected, ". . .when examining a new patient, read as little as possible of the old record before obtaining fresh evidence."

what is going on. When you find a particularly useful comment let the nurse who wrote it know. You will often find that useful comments in the notes increase. Similarly, social workers and nutritionists enter valuable information into the chart.

□ The Comprehensive History

When you are assigned a hospitalized patient you will usually be able to perform a Problem-Centered interview and *Comprehensive History* at the same time. You can proceed in two ways:

1. Follow the procedure described in previous chapters for the Problem-Centered interview.

2. Do a Comprehensive History, then sort out Problem-Centered data from *Health Promotion* data.

The first method has the advantage of preparing you for out-patient work in which you may not have time for a Comprehensive History. Also there are times when a hospitalized patient is too ill for a Comprehensive History, or may be about to leave for an x-ray or another procedure, and you lack time for more than a Problem-Centered interview. Try both ways: some of you may be comfortable with one approach and some with another. Whatever your choice, the key to being effective is to know the use of the information you are acquiring. Is it contributing to problem-solving or to health promotion?

□ REFERENCES

Gross F: The emperor's new clothes syndrome (letter). N Engl J Med 1971; 285:863.
Parrino TA, Villanueva AG: The principles and practice of morning report. JAMA 1986; 256:730–733.

CHAPTER 18

INTERVIEWING IN THE MEDICAL OFFICE

While much of your medical school interviewing experience is with hospital patients, most of the health care in the United States takes place in physicians' offices. (*Outpatient* or *ambulatory care* facilities, and *clinics* are roughly equivalent terms for *physicians' offices*, and will be used interchangeably.) Americans see their physicians three to four times a year, but are hospitalized only once in ten years (both statistics are averages). The office setting, in addition to providing care for most acute illnesses and long-term management for chronic illness, is ideal for the Health Promotion services of prevention and early detection of disease.

New methods of financing and controlling health care costs, such as the Diagnosis Related Group (DRG) prospective payment system and prepaid plans such as Health Maintenance Organizations (HMOs), place emphasis on minimizing hospitalization time by (1) early discharge of patients, and (2) Health Promotion services that keep people out of the hospital in the first place. This trend increases the amount of care provided in outpatient facilities and in the home. The more comfortable you are interviewing and examining patients outside of the hospital, the better prepared you will be for the realities of medical practice.

☐ Office Personnel

The *receptionist* is the first person a patient talks to on the phone and the first person the patient meets when coming to a physician's office. The receptionist (who may also be the nurse in a small office) welcomes patients, retrieves the patient's chart, tells the physician that the patient has arrived (and lets the patient know if a long delay is likely), schedules appointments, and handles payments. As the initial person to greet patients on the telephone as well as in person, the receptionist has a significant influence on many aspects of a physician's practice (Sawyer, 1985).

The *office nurse* or *nursing assistant* calls the patient from the reception room, measures vital signs (blood pressure, temperature, pulse, respiration and weight—although not always on each visit, depending on office policy), obtains blood or urine specimens if the physician has requested them prior to the examination, and escorts the patient to a room to wait for the physician.

Large ambulatory care facilities have other personnel. A *Nurse Practitioner* (NP) is a registered nurse (RN) who has had additional training in basic clinical tasks such as patient assessment (interviewing and physical examination), diagnosis and treatment of common illness, and expediting care for seriously ill persons. A *Physician's Assistant* (PA) has similar responsibilities. In some states NP's and PA's may write some prescriptions. Both function under the supervision of a physician, but the boundaries are blurred and state regulations vary.

A *Laboratory Technician* performs a variety of tests on blood and urine and prepares bacteriological specimens. Some technicians also take x-rays, although this role is increasingly performed by an x-ray technician.

The *Office/Business Manager* is responsible for the overall efficiency of the office as well as supervising fee collections and financial management.

Large clinics are multi-million dollar operations with pharmacists, physiotherapists, and mental health and patient education professionals, and they use a variety of support services such as computers and sophisticated communications.

□ Types of Office Practice

Solo practice—a single physician meeting all patient needs—is rapidly disappearing. Many physicians, especially specialists, practice alone, but they usually arrange with other physicians to share night and week-end responsibilities, and they make use of nearby consultants and support services.

Today most physicians practice in some type of *group practice*. The simplest type of group consists of individual practitioners who occupy one large group building, which also houses laboratory, x-ray, pharmacy, and other services. In such arrangements each physician keeps individual patient records and bills independently. True group practices involve the sharing of a common group of patients and a single billing system. Sharing of income and clinic expenses take a variety of forms. A group practice may offer primary care plus a variety of clinical specialities, or may be a single speciality group. Finally, outpatient facilities may be owned by physicians, by a nearby hospital, or by local, state or federal agencies. Large health care organizations and national chains are rapidly expanding operations in the outpatient area.

□ The Student in a Physician's Office

Physicians' offices are busy places. They care for large numbers of patients, and must generate substantial revenues. Your presence can complicate things. While the physician and staff may be delighted to have you present, they may also view you as someone who will slow down patient flow.

As soon as possible, discuss with the preceptor what is expected of you and how you can help. For example, you can save the medical staff time by writing up the visit (legibly) for the physician's review and signature. Helping with nursing tasks like escorting the patient from the reception room gives you the opportunity to observe the patient move about in a realistic setting, and provides you with experience in measuring vital signs.

Generally, your medical school has made adequate arrangements with office practitioners ahead of time, but sometimes an office situation does not work as well as expected. Be alert to difficulties. If there is a problem, and you feel comfortable talking about it with the preceptor, do so at an appropriate time. If you do not feel safe in this approach, discuss the situation with your medical school advisor.

□ The Office Team

Office practice is a team effort. The physician is just one member of a team; the nurse may be the person who makes the team function smoothly. Be sensitive to the nurses' needs. This is their turf, and you have the potential to disrupt things. Always clean an examination room after you have used it, removing soiled paper from the examination table and replacing it with fresh. Save socialization for times when no patients are in the office. Don't hesitate to ask for advice. Some nurses can be valuable teachers, but you must indicate your willingness to be taught.

□ Office Professionalism

Offices usually have a more relaxed atmosphere than do hospitals. This informality sometimes results in needless distress for patients. Many offices are small and patients may overhear and misinterpret what you are saying. Laughing, joking, and eating in clinical areas detract from the professional environment.

□ Interviewing in the Office

Talking with patients, whether in a hospital or an office, involves the same procedures discussed in *Chapter 16: Procedure Basics*. In the outpatient setting, however, some modifications are needed. Time is the limiting factor. Office visits are scheduled for as little as 5 or 10 minutes. The leisurely, comprehensive evaluation given the hospitalized patient is rarely practical in the clinic setting. The structure of the interview described in this text is adapted to these realities. The Problem-Centered interview serves both as a stand-alone history during a brief office visit and as the initial component of a complete database adaptable to patients in or out of the hospital. Some physicians use questionnaires to obtain a substantial part of the clinical information. Also, computer-based interviewing is beginning to appear (see *Unit VIII: Technical Supports*). Even without such aids, a database can be accumulated a little at a time during consecutive office visits.

Many patients seen in the office are there for a follow-up of an already diagnosed condition. In such circumstances you will need to review the patient's chart to become familiar with the diagnosis and current therapy. Such visits are brief; the office schedule doesn't allow you time to discuss the patient's history in depth.

□ Patient Comfort

One factor to consider (even though it may be out of your control) is patient comfort. In the interest of efficiency, some office practices ask the patient to undress and put on a gown before the interview and examination begins. Gowns are often flimsy paper, and most do not provide for a patient's modesty or warmth. Developing rapport under such circumstances is difficult. The practice of a few physicians who immediately place women with gyneco- logical complaints in a lithotomy position, even before the history taking has started, cannot be defended in any situation other than for a brief routine follow-up visit, and even then the practice discourages discussion of new problems the physicians has not anticipated.

□ History-taking by the Office Staff

The receptionist or office nurse may have entered in the chart the reason for the visit or a brief history of the Present Illness. Some members of the office staff know the patients so well, and are so trusted, that a few words accurately capture the essence of the patient's problem. A patient may reserve some concerns solely for the physician, however. Be prepared for the possibility that the problem may be different than the one listed in the chart. In any event, you will gain the greatest value from each patient if you resist the temptation to rely on the history taken by others—ask for yourself.

□ The Home Visit

A part of many office practices is a home visit. With growing emphasis on early discharge of hospital patients, home care is an increasingly important part of medical practice. Primary care physicians, particularly, include house calls, on a selective basis, as a part of their practice (Siwek, 1985). While calls are time-consuming, compared to an office visit, they provide an opportunity to learn more about a patient as a person than will a dozen office visits.

For some patients, such as those with a disabling or terminal illness, there may be no practical alternative to seeing a patient at home. (The role of a home visit in caring for the elderly is discussed in *Chapter 23: The Geriatric Patient.*) For an acutely ill patient with overwhelming social problems, such as no baby sitter or transportation, a home visit may be the only practical way to get the patient into the health care system. In many instances, initial assessment can be done by a Visiting Nurse, but a visit by a physician establishes rapport that results in the patient finding ways to come to the office for future needs.

Interviewing at home presents some special problems. The patient may not be able to speak freely because of the presence of others. Distractions like the family dog nipping at your leg, or a loud TV, are obstacles. Usually, however, assessment can be carried out quickly and effectively.

If there is a question about the urgency of a house call and the request has come from someone other than the patient, ask to speak to the patient. Often the quality of the patient's voice (paralanguage), as well as what the patient says, solves the problem. How someone talks on the phone may tell you how serious their illness is. You can tell, too, when the request for a home visit was not the patient's idea, but the result of the caller's anxiety.

☐ Telephone Medicine

Telephone medicine is a difficult clinical speciality. You must make diagnostic and therapeutic judgments without the benefit of the nonverbal information that is so valuable in a face-to-face interview. You cannot examine the patient, although the Review of Systems is a way to examine the patient with words. Following the *Fundamental Four* and *Sacred Seven* assists accurate data collection. As you acquire experience, your telephone diagnostic skills will become more intuitive (Sloane et al, 1985).

Knowing the caller, one of the benefits of continuity of care, makes medical decisions easier and more accurate.

Mr. Gilbert had significant heart disease, but minimized its existence through denial. One Tuesday afternoon he called. He apologized for interrupting because all he needed was a "bit of advice." He was having some chest pain ("I'm sure it is just indigestion") and wanted the name of a good antacid to get at a local drugstore. This was the first time in the many years that I had cared for him that he had called me about a medical question. My reaction was that he would not be calling if all that concerned him was indigestion. A brief Present Illness interview added the information that the pain at times radiated to the left shoulder, and that he was aware of palpitations. It was clear on the phone that he was having a severe angina attack. I told him it was essential that he come to the Emergency Room immediately. An EKG showed definite ischemia not present on previous EKG's. He was admitted to the hospital (over his protests that it would be a lot of unnecessary trouble); shortly thereafter he suffered a major myocardial infarction.

Establishing a reliable telephone communication channel is a prime requisite for a successful practice. A definite routine involving reliable access to the physician or designated nurse must be established so that the patient is not "tied to the phone" for hours awaiting a call. Breakdowns in telephone communication are a frequent source of patient dissatisfaction.

A brief note in a patient's chart about every telephone call, and your recommendations, is an essential part of telephone medicine. Also, a system for routine follow-up is valuable. Patients appreciate the concern, and the clinician learns the effectiveness of the recommended care. Also, a follow-up call provides a safety factor in case the situation proves to be more serious than initially estimated.

□ Office Records

You should know as much as possible about the patient before you walk into the examining room; trying to listen to the patient as you thumb through the record does not get the visit off to a good start. Experienced physicians arrive at the office in enough time to review all patients' charts at the beginning of each clinic session. This assists in planning for the best use of the doctor's time, and in obtaining tests, such as a blood count or a urinalysis, that are needed before seeing the patient.

Write up the chart entry immediately after seeing a patient, or if you are under extreme time pressure, jot down key data. Some physicians let large piles of records accumulate and then try to complete all of them at one sitting. Clinical notes entered days or weeks after the patient's visit are of questionable accuracy.

Keeping charts immediately available is as essential in a medical office as in a hospital unit. The clinic record must not leave the office for any reason. Nor should the record be left in the room with the patient if you have to step out. Patients have a right to know what is in their medical record, but not as an accidental event.

□ REFERENCES AND READINGS

Arbes S, Sawyer L: The role of the receptionist in general practice: A "dragon behind the desk?" Soc Sci Med 1985; 20:911–921.
Golden A, Grayson M, Bartlett E, Barker LR: The doctor-patient relationship: Communication and

patient education. In Barker, LR, Burton, JR, Zieve, PD: Principles of Ambulatory Medicine, ed 2. Baltimore, Williams & Wilkins, 1986, Chap 3.

Siwek J: House calls: Current status and rationale. Am Family Physician 1985; 31:169–174.

Sloane PP, Egelhoff C, Curtis P, et al: Physician decision making over the telephone. J Fam Pract 1985; 21:279–284.

Wassersug JD: What you will never learn unless you make house calls. Med Econ 1985; July 22:135–138.

CHAPTER 19

THE INTERVIEW AS THERAPY AND PATIENT EDUCATION

The interview serves not only for diagnosis and health promotion, but also for patient education and therapy.

☐ Patient Education

Following the interview and physical examination the patient wants to know what was found and what the future holds in terms of further testing, treatment, and likely outcome (prognosis). For many conditions, especially chronic diseases, therapy involves providing a substantial amount of information about the nature of the patient's illness, and negotiating about treatment (Greenfield, 1985). Sometimes only a few words of instruction are necessary, but extensive research has demonstrated that clinicians seriously misjudge what patients know and understand about their illnesses (Evans and Haynes, 1984). Furthermore, few patients have the courage to ask questions. The result is often misunderstanding about diagnosis and treatment, commonly leading to the failure of the patient to carry out the recommended therapy. Also, incomplete or inaccurate understanding results in unnecessary anxiety. A deliberate effort to monitor patients' understanding of their condition and to create an environment that encourages questions is an essential part of effective care.

Patients are now, much more than in the past, urged to take responsibility for their own care (Fletcher, 1985). Commercial interests have rushed to meet the need for everything from do-it-yourself pregnancy testing kits to comprehensive nutritional plans. Millions of persons participate in fitness programs.

While the self-care movement in general is a healthy one, professional advice helps patients avoid worthless or dangerous self-care activities.

Giving patients information about their condition is one step in creating a working partnership. Some physicians give their patients a copy of the chart entry for each visit, or dictate a special note for the patient. Computer-based records are ideal for this purpose. Patients can be given summaries of common illnesses; these can be written in nontechnical language and kept in a loose-leaf binder, or they can be copied and then individualized notes can be added as necessary (Griffith, 1983). Also, many pharmaceutical companies prepare for free distribution helpful patient education materials.

Patients should also carry in their wallet or purse a complete health care summary in case of illness away from the usual source of care. Small, easily carried cards are available or can be made. You should encourage patients with serious conditions that may render them unable to give information in an emergency to wear a clearly visible Medic Alert* warning pendant or bracelet.

Patient education is a growing part of comprehensive care. It is good medical practice. It encourages intelligent cooperation in therapy, and contributes to the patient's self-esteem and personal growth. The economic and time pressures of a busy clinical practice invite omission of patient education, but the few minutes needed to assure that patients understand their diagnosis and treatment is often the factor that makes the difference between success and failure of care.

☐ Informed Consent

A special case of patient information is the legal concept of informed consent. Patients should understand their condition and its therapy; the question is: In how much detail? Informed consent, taken to its extremes, would require that the physician explain in detail every possible complication associated with treatment as a prerequisite for the patient's decision whether or not to accept care. The fact is that patients neither want nor can understand the more technical aspects of their therapy. Most patients trust their physicians as advisors who will make the best decision possible on their behalf. "Reasonable" explanations are now accepted as all that is required. "Reasonable," of course, requires good judgment. If, for example, a man is advised to have prostate surgery that will probably leave him impotent, the decision should be discussed in detail. But to also tell him that there exists a chance of fatal hemorrhage and other complications during surgery, however remote the possibilities, serves no purpose other than confusing the patient and perhaps providing an overanxious

---

*Patients who participate in the Medic Alert system complete an extensive personal record form that is available by telephone to emergency medical personnel 24 hours a day. The Medic Alert pendant or bracelet names the patient's major problem as well as giving the patient's identification number. Medic Alert, a nonprofit organization, can be reached at Turlock, CA 95380.

surgeon with a sense of protection against a lawsuit. Several references listed at the end of this chapter discuss informed consent in detail.

□ Therapeutic Aspects

Although the *Fundamental Four* serve primarily a diagnostic purpose, some of the information has implications for therapy: co-existing medical conditions, medications the patient is already taking, the patient's work and the home situation frequently enter into decisions about the kind of therapy that will be appropriate for a new illness.

□ Therapeutic Interview Techniques

Some of the interviewing techniques described in *Unit IV: Communication Techniques* have therapeutic potential, and a few risks.

Focused Reflection brings to the patient's attention some issue that has come up during the interview that you feel merits elaboration.

"When I asked about your family, you seemed upset when mentioning your son who still lives at home."

"You have been late to your last three appointments—is there a problem about coming here?"

"You don't sound very enthusiastic about being retired."

These responses present an opportunity for the patient to discuss the issue further. If the patient doesn't elaborate, you must decide whether to pursue the matter with direct questioning, or to just note it for discussion in the future.

Interpretation is a generalization based on a number of specific happenings you feel may be linked.

"With so many unsatisfactory things happening, I wonder if you are having doubts about your decision to go to medical school."

"While you haven't come right out and said so, I get the impression that your marriage is in real difficulty."

Interpretations are tools of psychotherapists. Whether to introduce them in a nonpsychotherapeutic setting depends on your ability to deal with the underlying issues.

□ Support: Just Being There

Support counters the loneliness that accompanies illness by demonstrating that you are an ally. Just being involved is therapeutic. The power of a professional's presence is one of the forces behind the effectiveness of Medicine Men and other folk healers. If you, or someone in your family, has been acutely ill, you may remember the sudden lessening of tension when the physician appeared, or even just established contact by phone. Sometimes the "laying on of hands" meets the patient's needs.

> *Mrs. B was a 28-year-old housewife with progressive multiple sclerosis. I saw her monthly, and performed a brief neurological examination each time—I'm not sure why, as there was nothing that could be done to alter the fundamental disease.*
>
> *One summer I was to be away at the time of her regular visit, and arranged for a colleague to see her. When I next saw the patient, she expressed dissatisfaction with the other physician. She said, "I know there isn't anything really that can be done, but at least you examine me. He didn't."*

Also, a sense of support emerges just with sharing a problem with an understanding, interested, and professionally trained person. Explaining an illness to a clinician helps the patient look objectively at a situation, perhaps for the first time. New facts are remembered, associations between events and situations recognized, and concerns are seen in a more balanced perspective.

Finally, some patient problems involve distorted ideas, unrealistic attitudes and excessive emotional responses. Many such problems are best treated with words and appropriate emotional support, sometimes supplemented with medication. The "talking cure" is the primary activity of psychiatrists and psychologists, but these mental health specialists care for only a very small number of all persons who can benefit from professional help. Every clinician, regardless of speciality, practices psychotherapy to some degree during every patient interaction.

☐ Reassurance

Reassurance goes a step beyond support; it signals that you are involved and taking action that will address the problem as effectively as possible. One form of reassurance is by giving information. Patients often are more upset about what they think is the significance of a condition than the condition itself. Today, health advice and information, ranging from excellent to very bad, are freely given. Misinformation is common, and guilt, shame, or a vivid imagination can create a state of fear or panic. Providing authoritative information is often all that is needed to put a patient's mind at ease. Sexual concerns are a frequent focus of unwarranted anxiety, as discussed in *Chapter 24: The Sexual History.*

Serious diseases, such as cancer, are another area in which giving information is an essential part of caring for a patient. "Cancer," to the average person, signifies a fatal disease. Not everyone knows that there are all sorts of cancers, some no more serious than a bad cold. A basal cell cancer of the skin, for example, is usually curable with simple removal. If, however, all the patient hears is the word "cancer," without being told that this kind of skin cancer, appropriately treated, is 100 percent curable, anxiety or depression is an understandable reaction. To further complicate such a situation, many people are reluctant to express their fears, feeling that to do so is a sign of weakness. As in many other situations involving what the patient considers to be unacceptable emotions, you have to take the initiative to discover what the patient is unable to express.

Understanding what the patient is experiencing is another component of reassurance. When you actively listen to both the facts and the emotions of a patient's illness, the patient knows you have a grasp of the entire situation. An example of how reassurance results from this kind of understanding is the case of the young woman with Hodgkin's disease described in *Chapter 8: Risk Factors in Diagnosis and Treatment.* Comments like:

"I can share your feeling of frustration."

"That's a very understandable response to this sort of situation."

"The symptoms you are describing are very common in this condition."

communicate that you are familiar with what the patient is experiencing and know what to do to next.

A part of this kind of understanding is accepting what the patient is experiencing, however, irrational it may seem. A person who anticipates not being taken seriously, or ridicule, may not have the courage to share with others frightening thoughts and feelings. Sometimes just a few words are genuinely reassuring.

Mr. Sanders, a 45-year-old man who prided himself on his robust health, finally had to admit that the increasingly severe chest pain merited attention. His wife called an ambulance. The Emergency Room physician told him that he was in the early stages of a heart attack and needed to be admitted to the hospital. Never having been in the hospital before, the patient felt out of control and frightened. The orderly taking the patient to the coronary care unit on a stretcher noticed his apprehension. He put his hand on Mr. Sanders' shoulder and said, "Now Mr. Sanders, we take care of patients with heart attacks all the time, and they do just fine."

The patient said later that the sense that he wasn't "the first" somehow brought him a sense of relief and comfort.

The patient added a touch of humor in relating the ambulance ride. The vehicle was one that had frosted glass windows with an etched cross in the center. "You know those windows with the crosses?" he asked. I bet you don't know what is on the inside." I said I did not. "Well—on one side is a MasterCard decal, and on the other side a VISA decal."

In a fine text on the kinds of psychological support easily incorporated into any medical practice, *The Twenty Minute Hour*, Castelnuovo-Tedesco (1965) summarizes that people feel reassured when they feel understood, when their own understanding increases as a result of a comment the doctor has made, when they feel accepted, and finally

..a person feels reassured if he is not overly reassured. The dosage must be right. Since total reassurance is impossible to give (or receive), enthusiastic statements generally are useless and only convince the patient that the doctor has no understanding of the problem.

☐ Belief Systems

Many physicians recognize that belief systems—feelings about God, good and evil, guilt and forgiveness—play an important role in the health and disease of their patients. Solid experimental evidence demonstrates that the immune system can be conditioned by mental phenomena, a finding that helps explain why some people fall ill at times of psychological stress, and why others overcome seemingly hopeless medical conditions (Ader, 1981). Peck (1978), a psychoanalyst, viewing religion in terms of a world view rather than membership in an organized religious group, believes that different world views lead to different life patterns. A world seen as inherently chaotic, hostile or intolerant of any error, or as a ruthless context for survival, leads people to a live a different kind of life than does a world seen as nurturing, forgiving, or purposeful. He writes:

There are all manner of different world views that people have...And it is essential that therapists arrive at this knowledge, for the world view of patients is always an essential part of their problems, and a correction in their world view is necessary for their cure.

Most physicians do not engage patients at such a fundamental level of understanding, but there are times in any type of practice where helping the patient achieve a sustaining spiritual philosophy has an important influence on the medical outcome.

□ Giving Advice

Giving advice is tempting. It fulfills our wish to be helpful, and it does our ego good to play the role of sage. But giving advice carries with it responsibility. If something goes wrong with a course of action you endorse, you may be blamed for the a poor outcome. But whether the outcome is favorable or unfavorable, you have deprived the patient of an opportunity for personal growth. For a person to benefit from a significant personal decision, the person must have created it and "own it."

A friendly neutrality best helps the patient reach a decision. Think of yourself as a catalyst, giving encouragement that problems can be solved, providing relevant information, and asking questions that develop options for the person to consider. Only rarely will you have to take a stand—for example, if the patient's intent is obviously harmful or dangerous. Finally, if you find yourself compelled to judge or give advice, you may be unconsciously acting out your problems through the patient. This subject is explored more fully in *Chapter 20: Difficult Relationships.*

□ Pseudo-advice: Blaming the Patient

Patients who get better under our care are good for our self-esteem. None of us like to care for a patient who is not improving despite our best efforts. One way out of our discomfort is a false kind of advice which returns full responsibility for the outcome of a condition to the patient:

"If you are going to continue to smoke, you cannot expect your asthma to get better."

"Your weight won't go down until you follow the diet I gave you."

These responses, whether said gently or in a scolding way, rarely tell patients anything they don't already know. Such advice, however, weakens rapport and lessen the chances of eventual success. If you feel unable to work with patients with problems such as smoking, drinking, or overeating, transfer the patient to a practitioner who can tolerate the personal frustrations that accompany caring for patients with difficult-to-cure problems.

□ The Student's Role in Therapy and Patient Education

As you work with a patient through a diagnostic evaluation, it is natural to want to participate in therapy. Providing advice and patient education is one of the pleasures of clinical care. It signifies that the diagnostic work-up has been successful and that a plan of therapy has been reached. As a medical student, however, you must recognize that this aspect of care is the responsibility of the patient's attending physician. To offer the patient advice and recommend therapy, without the attending physician's prior knowledge and approval, could be a disservice to both the patient and the patient's physician, and could possibly involve you in disciplinary action.

Sometimes the "attending" elects a plan of action that differs from what your teachers and readings recommend. When this happens, it is appropriate to tactfully discuss the question of optimal care on rounds. Often there are several equally effective approaches to the same problem. Many times the physician's choice of therapy is based on having known the patient for years and understanding what will work best given the patient's unique circumstance. If, however, you should find yourself in a situation where you are very uncomfortable about a preceptor's action and do not feel safe in discussing your concerns with the physician, it is appropriate to discuss the matter with your medical school advisor.

In most instances, your participation in therapy and patient education will be welcomed, and the patient's doctor will be delighted to delegate to you the task of explaining to the patient the nature of the diagnosis and the plans for therapy.

☐ REFERENCES AND READINGS

Ader R (ed): Psychoneuroimmunology. New York, Academic Press, 1981.

Bartlett EE, Stephens GG: Patient education. *In* Taylor RB: Family Medicine: Principles and Practice, ed 2. New York, Springer-Verlag, 1983, Ch 28, pp 332–337.

Castelnuovo-Tedesco P: The Twenty-Minute Hour. Boston, Little, Brown & Co, 1965.

Curran WJ: Informed consent in malpractice cases. A turn toward reality. N Engl J Med 1986;314:82–85.

Evans CE, Haynes RB: Patient compliance. *In* Rakel RE (ed): Textbook of Family Practice, ed 3. Philadelphia, WB Saunders Co, 1984, Ch 27, pp 325–337.

Fletcher DJ: Self-care: How to help patients share responsibility for their health. Postgraduate Med 1985;78:213–223.

Greenfield S, Kaplan S, Ware JE: Expanding patient involvement in care: Effects on patient outcomes. Ann Intern Med 1985;102:520–528.

Griffith HW: Instructions for Patients, ed 4. Philadelphia, WB Saunders Co, In preparation.

Griffith HW, Attarian P, Harrison WT: Patient health education. *In* Taylor RB: Family Medicine: Principles and Practice, ed 2. New York, Springer-Verlag, 1983, Ch 97, pp 1835–1848.

Holinger PC, Tubesing DA: Models of health and wholeness. J Religion and Health 1979;18:203–211.

Katz J: The Silent World of Doctor and Patient. New York, The Free Press/Macmillan, 1984.

Litz CW, Meisel A, Zerubavel E, et al: Informed Consent: A Study of Decisionmaking in Psychiatry. New York, Guilford Press, 1984.

Miller G, Shank JC: Patient education: Comparative effectiveness by means of presentation. J Fam Pract 1985;22:178–181.

Peck MS: The Road Less Traveled. New York, Simon and Schuster, 1978.

Sherlock R: Reasonable men and sick human beings. Am J Med 1986;80:2–4.

Weed LL: Your Health Care and How to Manage It. Essex Junction, VT, Essex Publishing Company, revised printing 1978.

UNIT VI

SPECIAL INTERVIEWS

CHAPTER 20

DIFFICULT RELATIONSHIPS

Most doctors and most patients get along well with each other. An occasional patient, however, brings out in us feelings and behaviors we hardly recognize as our own. These reactions may be harsh and negative—anger, rudeness, withdrawal, fear, depression, even hatred; or they may be inappropriately positive—excessive concern, ingratiation, even seduction. Either way a disturbance in the doctor-patient relationship is taking place, which clashes with our wish to help people and with our sense of professionalism.

Discussion of physicians' counter-therapeutic reactions to their patients usually focus on *patients'* qualities that create the difficulty. The patient is labeled "difficult," or worse. A much-discussed article in *The New England Journal of Medicine* described the *hateful* patient, "one whom most physicians would dread to treat." A more balanced view, however, will acknowledge the fact that we as clinicians unconsciously play a part in relationships that do not go well. In most instances, counter-therapeutic reactions are the result of certain kinds of inappropriate *interactions* between physician and patient—both persons contribute to the difficulty. Elements of each one's personality find a receptor in the personality of the other. Each receives some emotional "payoff" from the other, even though neither benefits in the long run.

Frequently, too, *situational factors*—constraints and circumstances in the health care delivery process, or in the personal lives of doctor or patient—intensify the counter-therapeutic reaction. This chapter will look at each of these factors in the counter-therapeutic relationship: the patient, the doctor, and the situational circumstances.

Just how you respond when you experience uncomfortable feelings with a patient depends on how well you know your patient—and yourself. "Difficult" patients need not be a cause of negative feelings if you can look beneath the surface and understand what the stresses of illness and the medical care process have activated in the person you are trying to help and in yourself. Out of conflict may emerge greater maturity for both of you. Indeed, sometimes you can even find humor in caring for a "difficult patient."

Every clinic has a few "regulars" who drink too much. Ours came in one day, without an appointment, in his usual unsteady state. What was different was that he had driven to the clinic although he lived only a short distance away (but on a busy street).

After taking care of his medical problem, I told him I wanted to drive him in his car back home. He accepted the offer, and said no more until I was about to walk back to the clinic. Then, with profuse thanks he said, "Isn't there something I can do for you—let me give you a ride to the clinic?"

Most of the clues to the difficult situation, and its successful resolution, emerge during the interview. Both the verbal and nonverbal content communicate when trouble is brewing. The interview is also the tool with which the difficulty can be minimized or resolved.

☐ Patient Characteristics

Most patients' contact with the medical profession is brief, and peripheral to the important areas of their lives. "Problem patients" are different. Their relationship with their physician is more substantial. It has more dimensions. Sometimes the doctor and the doctor's staff are a patient's only source of human contact, interest, advice, or outlet for bottled-up feelings. A "visit to the doctor" is an important occasion, which provides brief but valued relief from an otherwise isolated or depressing life.

Attempts to classify these patients (Groves, 1978; Klein et al, 1982; Smith, 1984) include characteristics such as:

- [ ] Emotional/Unreasonable/Hysterical.
- [ ] Highly dependent.
- [ ] Passive-aggressive.
- [ ] Controlling/Independent.
- [ ] Ingratiating/Flattering/Seducing.
- [ ] Manipulative/Deceitful/Dishonest/Fraudulent.
- [ ] Uncooperative/Undisciplined.
- [ ] Medical system abusers.
- [ ] Demanding/Complaining.
- [ ] Low pain tolerance/Whiny.
- [ ] Self-destructive (substance abuser/smoker/suicidal).
- [ ] Health faddist/"Know-it-all."

These characteristics are, to varying degrees, qualities for which the patient can be held "accountable." Rightly or wrongly, we see these behaviors as under the patient's control, behaviors for which the patient is "responsible," and for which the patient can be "blamed."

Other patients are usually not thought to be responsible for their situations, but they stress and frustrate their caretakers nevertheless. Such patients may be considered:

- [ ] Ignorant/Low intelligence/Mentally retarded.
- [ ] Psychotic.
- [ ] Terminally ill.
- [ ] Undiagnosable.
- [ ] Victims of tragic life circumstances.

□ Practitioner Characteristics

Next, let's look at the other side of the coin—the physician's characteristics that have the potential for conflict when interacting with some patients. Such qualities might include:

- [ ] Scientific/Objective/Reasonable.
- [ ] Unemotional/Detached.
- [ ] Overly Responsible/Conscientious.
- [ ] Perfectionistic.
- [ ] Controlling.

☐ Dependent/Need to be needed.
☐ Overly cautious/Avoid harming.
☐ Seeking status among peers and in the community.
☐ Idealistic/Altruistic/Self-sacrificing.
☐ Self-sufficient/Self-reliant/Disciplined.
☐ Rescuing/Heroic.
☐ Highly ethical/Moral.
☐ Needing personal time for family and recreation.

Interaction defines the meaning in any specific doctor-patient relationship. Whether or not we find a particular patient to be "difficult" is determined by the interaction of our unique personhood with the patient's unique personhood. Sometimes a patient who interacts poorly with one physician gets along very well with another. Some patients are charming with their physician, but rude and demanding with the physician's staff, just as a person may be different at work than at home.

For example, consider the interaction likely to develop between a dependent patient and a physician who needs to be needed.

Dr. Carney was a fine internist. The most notable thing about Dr. Carney, however, was his universal willingness to be helpful. He saw patients anytime they wanted to be seen, including hours when the clinic was closed except for emergencies. If another member of the staff needed to trade an on-call night, Dr. Carney was the first one asked because he almost never refused. Inevitably, he was taken advantage of by patients and staff, all the while enjoying his too well-earned reputation as being "a nice guy."

For whatever reason, Dr. Carney fulfilled important emotional needs by being of service to his patients and staff. He had a need to be needed. But his patients paid a hidden price. Many, overly dependent to begin with, became even more dependent on Dr. Carney. They never had a chance to grow, at least within that part of their life involving their health care. When physicians like Dr. Carney retire, they leave a lot of patients who are unlikely to find another physician willing to be as generous as was Dr. Carney.

☐ Situational Difficulties

Added to conflict-causing personal qualities are situational stresses which, while arising outside the clinical setting, intrude into the professional relationship. At times, elements such as these dominate the health care interaction:

☐ Time pressures/Work load.
☐ Physician's inability to obtain for the patient the care thought to be necessary.
☐ Administrative overcontrol/Paperwork.

□ Physician's personal stresses: physical or mental illness, substance abuse, family stresses.

Patients bring a similar collection of background stresses into the clinical relationship. They may not have the funds or insurance to afford care. Dealing with public care agencies may leave a person about to see the doctor exhausted and irritable. Patients may be under intolerable stresses at home or at work.

A 50-year-old tailor, a recent immigrant from Europe who was barely able to support his large family, was admitted to the hospital because of pneumonia. The acute illness responded well to antibiotics, but repeat X-ray films revealed an underlying process, which proved to be active tuberculosis. When the patient was told of this condition and the need for prolonged rest as a necessary part of tuberculosis treatment, he became quite angry and demanded to be released from the hospital. He had a family to support, he said, and they were his first and only important obligation.

□ Mechanism of Conflict

To detail all the factors that contribute to difficult relationships would go beyond the scope of this essay into psychology and sociology. The brief tabulation presented, based on the above factors, suggests how conflicts arise when a physician characteristic and a patient or situational characteristic clash.

Patient	Doctor
Health faddist	Scientific objectivity
Dependent	Self-sufficient
Independent	Controlling
Seductive	Needing affection
Complaining	Self-reliant
Smoker	Non-smoker
Without funds	Idealism
Complex problem	Mastery/Control
High risk	Safety/Avoiding harm

□ Nonadaptive Responses

When conflicts develop, we may respond in ways that control the surface manifestations, but do not solve the underlying problem. We may seek to diminish or eliminate our contact with the patient, or we may move towards the patient. Some of these reactions may be expressed by:

Decreasing Contact

☐ Avoiding the patient and family.
☐ Not returning phone calls.
☐ Emotional withdrawal.
☐ Intellectualization.
☐ "Blaming the victim."
☐ Ridicule/Belittlement.

Increasing Contact

☐ Loving/Affectionate/Seductive.
☐ Overly responsible.
☐ Prolonging care.
☐ Infantalizing.
☐ Ingratiating.
☐ Excessively conscientious.
☐ Overly cautious ("defensive medicine").
☐ Overly solicitous/Hovering/Excessive follow-up.
☐ Lecturing and Moralizing.
☐ Punishing/Depriving.

Our personal conflicts can interfere with a wholesome, enjoyable practice in other ways. Substance abuse, unless recognized and treated early, is devastating to a physician's professional and personal life. Financial insecurity may result in performing unnecessary surgery or expensive procedures. Unresolved sexual concerns may take the form of inappropriately detailed sexual histories. Someone whose family background was humble may unconsciously cultivate a practice of executives and VIP's.

Medical conditions with strong *moral* implications frequently cause difficulty. Abortion, homosexuality, substance abuse, or contraception may interfere with clinical objectivity. Because of the widespread public discussion of these areas, most practitioners are aware of their attitudes about such issues and can separate personal values from professional service. Sometimes, however, reason loses out to strong feelings, which take the form of avoidance, rudeness, or lecturing and other forms of moral persuasion. The physician may unconsciously choose to remain blind to difficult-to-deal-with problems by ignoring subtle evidence and not asking appropriate questions, thus indirectly perpetuating the difficulties (Anderson, 1986).

☐ Internalized Negative Responses

Beyond the stresses that manifest themselves in the doctor-patient interaction are those the professional keeps inside:

□ Guilt.
□ Rationalization.
□ Depression.
□ Professional isolation.
□ Over-identification with patients and their problems.

Much of the stress of practice, and the growing syndrome of "burnout," can be traced to dissonance between valid but incompatible values. The conscientious physician, for example, may find not enough hours in the day to be invariably responsible to patients and also have personal time for family and recreation. Compromise, making either/or choices, and tolerating uncertainty are skills not always learned in medical school; we have difficulty meeting conflicting demands in a world where less-than-satisfactory answers must sometimes be accepted (see *Chapter 11: Uncertainty*).

□ Recognizing Counter-Therapeutic Reactions

Given the theory—how does it work in practice? The key is recognizing that something isn't right; that you need to stop, take a look at what is going on, and dissect out the various elements. The problem may be with the patient, within yourself, in the situational circumstances, or sometimes all three. Here are some of the warning signals, the yellow lights, that say proceed with caution until the problem is identified and under as much control as possible:

Preoccupation. Thinking about the patient at times when ordinarily your mind would be on other matters. The thoughts may be pleasant or unpleasant, but distorted and intrusive.

Anticipation. Looking forward to the patient's next visit eagerly, or with dread. Either way there is a compulsive quality to the expectations.

Avoidance. One way or another, we either cancel, or think of canceling, the patient's next visit. This reaction commonly is quite unconscious—for example, making conflicting appointments. Another form of avoidance is using excessive control during the interview to ensure that uncomfortable issues do not arise.

Making Exceptions. Making special arrangements for a particular patient in areas such as scheduling appointments; increasing, decreasing, or eliminating fees; accommodating requests ordinarily not granted; giving, inviting, or accepting inappropriate gifts.

Intense Emotions. Guilt, anger, fear, love, hate: Intense feelings of any kind are signals that a personal issue is distorting our perception of the patient.

☐ Labeling Patients

Making premature or incorrect generalizations is one factor in development of the difficult patient relationship. Generalizations are necessary; life would be impossible if we had to assume that every person was unique and totally unlike anyone we had ever met before. The trouble comes when we form a judgment about a person on the basis of too little information. Once a patient has been labeled as a certain type, such as "dependent," "passive-aggressive," or "depressive," a vicious spiral between doctor and patient begins which confirms the stereotype. A "dependent" patient, for example, quickly finds the doctor attempting to escape being depended upon; intensified attempts to be cared for are met with increasing withdrawal by the practitioner. After a number of cycles, an uneasy equilibrium is reached and maintained, sometimes for years. What is true for the person with dependent needs is true for other kinds of "difficult" patients—people who make their way in the world with behaviors that control, manipulate, threaten, bully, plead, seduce, flatter, or any of the other negative terms that characterize persons who many health care providers would prefer to avoid.

☐ The Fallacy of Mistaken Identity

Another element in counter-therapeutic reactions might be called *mistaken identity**—unconsciously mistaking the patient for someone important in your personal life. In other words, transferring to a patient the feelings and attitudes that developed in a completely different setting and involved an altogether different person. The process sometimes activates strong emotions which exert their influence on how you relate to the patient—positively or negatively. A patient with terminal cancer may, for example, reactivate feelings you have about some close family member who died with the same disease. A demanding patient may remind you of a demanding parent—only now *you* are the one with power.

Or you may identify with a patient. For example, you may readily identify with a graduate student who is deep in debt and working long hours to get through college. Such situations have the potential for forming a protecting or rescuing relationship. Or someone who appears to have been victimized by some social injustice may remind you of times when you felt unjustly treated. Some of your reactions may in fact be similar to those of your patient; this is

---

*The terms *transference* and *counter-transference* used by psychotherapists are roughly equivalent to mistaken identity.

the basis of helpful empathy. The danger is that a patient may react very differently than you would in the same circumstances; what would have been helpful to you may not help the patient.

Mistaken identify cannot be avoided. What is needed is the ability to recognize when it is happening—the clues mentioned above are helpful signals—and to not act inappropriately. In fact, once attuned to the process, you will better understand yourself. If, for example, you find yourself unaccountably irritated by a person from a minority group, this may be a clue to a long-buried prejudice.

The process of mistaken identity works both ways. You may remind a patient of someone else, for better or worse. A patient you meet for the first time will have to rely on pre-existing judgments about doctors in general. Someone whose past experiences with practitioners have been hurtful will anticipate that you, too, will be hurtful. To the degree that you are authoritarian, the patient will activate attitudes based on experience with other authorities, like a parent, priest, school principal, or judge. If past experiences have taught the patient that authorities can be trusted, your patient will trust you from the onset.

Just as inappropriate reactions on your part provide you with new insights about yourself, similar reactions by your patients will tell you a lot about that patient. Someone who unreasonably criticizes you may do the same towards everyone, which can be useful diagnostic information. Some psychiatrists deliberately hold self-disclosure to a minimum to allow the patient's past patterns to emerge and be modified during therapy.

□ Managing The Difficult Relationship

□ COMMUNICATION

Most problems with professional relationships are solved in the course of daily professional activities. *Communication* is the common thread.

Personal sharing with respected peers opens up new approaches. Just as patients gain insight from explaining a problem to you, you can benefit by talking over a situation with a colleague.

Patient Care Conferences in which patient management problems are openly and honestly presented to your colleagues take courage, but are a part of professional growth. Discovering your shortcomings in such a forum does not diminish your status—quite the contrary.

Referring patients about whose care you feel uncomfortable. There are always situations in which insight and understanding fail to establish a good relationship. Both you and the patient are better off if you transfer the care of such patients to someone else. Some physicians feel that referring patients is an admission of weakness and "hang on" no matter how clear the indications that the relationship isn't going to work. Dimsdale (1984) cites instances in which difficult relationships lead not only to emotional distress but also to failure to diagnose obvious disease.

Regarding problems of mistaken identity, past generalizations blend with present reality. You and most of your patients will be sufficiently aware and flexible to keep past experiences in the background. The more they get to know you and you get to know them, the more accurate will be your perceptions of each other.

Don't overlook the value of simple, straightforward questions like "We really don't seem to get along very well, do we? What do you think is the problem?"

Sometimes a clinician can help the patient gain insight. Some of the communication techniques described in *Chapter 19: The Interview as Therapy and Patient Education* can initiate the process. How far to go with psychotherapy is a function of the clinician's experience in dealing with psychological difficulties. Many such patients are competently handled by primary care physicians without extensive psychotherapy training.

Some patients, unfortunately, maintain fixed attitudes, positive and negative, and cannot see you for who you are. Sooner or later, their fantasized concept of you leads to disappointment or conflict. Beneath these behaviors, however, are unmet human needs whose expression is distorted and often unacceptable to those persons who are important to them. This is evident in a primary care practice where continuity provides the repeated contacts for true feelings and behavior to emerge. If you can deflect anger and not respond in kind, you will at the very least not reinforce the patient's negative behavior, and at best may find ways to tap that part of the person which is capable of mature giving and receiving.

□ SELF-KNOWLEDGE

Knowing your own needs, strengths, and vulnerabilities is an essential part of managing difficult situations. Honestly explore your personal priorities, including the role you want medicine to play in your life. Think through the practice situation that will be right for you. Evolving forms of group practice HMO's and reimbursement mechanisms, such as the Diagnosis-Related Groups (DRG), have important implications for the doctor-patient relationship. If personal problems seem to defy self-analysis (as they often do), discuss them with a friend or a professional advisor. The time to avoid becoming an "impaired physician" is when a problem first surfaces.

□ FINDING PRACTICAL SOLUTIONS

Imbedded in some counter-productive situations are elements, perhaps not obvious ones, that can lessen their negative impact. Be creative. With ingenuity, answers can be found. If the problem is administrative red-tape, perhaps a call from you will straighten things out. Look for new perspectives. The intensity and scope of medicine sometimes blind us to fresh approaches to the problems of illness and daily living. Much depends on attitude. If a condition is labeled hopeless and nothing further attempted, then the prediction becomes self-confirming.

□ Common Difficult Relationships

□ HOSTILITY

Sooner or later you will encounter hostility from a patient. The patient may be rude, demeaning, sarcastic, challenging, or order you out of the room (or worse). Returning the anger is a natural response, but also terminates the relationship. No one wins when both persons are angry. Instead, try to understand *why* the patient is angry. Sometimes a patient's anger has nothing to do with you; you just walk into a situation at the wrong time.

My newly assigned patient clearly was not in a good mood. "Take that black bag and get out!" he said as soon as I introduced myself and explained why I was there. There was obviously no point in arguing, but as I started to leave I managed to ask why he was so angry with me since he'd never seen me before. He replied, "If you had spent all morning in X-ray with no breakfast, then the machine wouldn't work right, and finally you were sent back here without the X-ray and without any lunch being saved—how would you feel?" "I'd be mad as hell," I said as I started to leave. "Right—that's how I feel." Then after a pause he said, "Now, what can I do for you?"
I got him a lunch and later returned to complete my assignment. We became good friends during his hospital stay.

Despite your best efforts and sense of professionalism, you will get openly angry at a patient.

It was the first time I took night call for the clinic I'd joined. At 3 a.m. the phone rang. The caller, a young woman, described her symptoms—a slight fever, sore throat and sneezing. I interrupted her and said with all the sarcasm I could manage, "And you call me at this time of night with the symptoms of a common cold!!"
After a long pause it was obvious that she was crying. I managed to get her to tell me more about her concerns. The situation: she was calling from the airport where she had just landed after a visit home. She was 10 weeks' pregnant, and had had eight hours on the plane to think about her mother's final warning: "Now, when you get home, be sure to get care for that fever—you remember that Barbara down the street with the malformed child had the very same thing when she was pregnant, and she just ignored it."

While there are times when everyone is better off when you express your anger, this was not one of them. The patient's anxiety and 3 a.m. call were understandable. There is almost always a good reason for the patient's behavior if you take the time to ask a few questions. People, as a rule, do not go about deliberately making physicians' lives difficult. But they may trigger anger because of preoccupation with their own problems. A Golden Rule of professional behavior is this:

Before reacting in anger at something a patient does or says, search for the reason underlying the patient's actions, and why you have become upset.

If you ask questions, rather than respond angrily, you will learn a lot about people, and about yourself. If you find yourself chronically angry, of course, then you need to search for deeper reasons within your own personality.

□ THE OVERLY TALKATIVE PATIENT

There is an aggressive quality about overly talkative patients. They have a controlling or dominating effect on the interviewer. One type of overly talkative patient is the obsessional person who insists on giving a highly detailed account of his or her illness. Guard against overuse of facilitating nods, gestures, or phrases. Ask specific questions early in the interview. Limit a show of interest when the patient supplies trivial detail, but show interest when the patient provides pertinent information. You may have to interrupt when sufficient information has been provided and ask another direct question to keep the interview focused. Some patients, however, cannot be hurried; you will just have to relax and accept the situation as gracefully as possible.

Another type of over-talkativeness is encountered in the poorly organized patient who rambles. Interrupt the patient who wanders and refocus attention on relevant material. A mental status examination may be indicated.

A third type of talkative patient exhibits a chattering quality which betrays underlying anxiety. A reassuring or supportive comment regarding the patient's evident anxiety is sometimes sufficient to calm the patient; if not, see if you can uncover the source of the anxiety.

□ THE CONFUSED OR FORGETFUL PATIENT

Most confused patients are easily identified as needing special care and a protective environment. Some patients with chronic brain disease, however, have so well adapted to a gradually increasing cognitive impairment that their deficits are not noticed. When the stress of illness, potent medications, or hospitalization occurs, their adjustment collapses. Some confused persons find that being overly nice and compliant is the best strategy to keep their world under control. Others, unable to comprehend what is happening, feel threatened, and become belligerent. At that point they are classified as *difficult.*

Performing the simple mental status examination explained in *Chapter 16: Procedure Basics*, if you think to do it, will clarify the situation.

Forgetting, particularly events in the recent past, often accompanies chronic brain impairment. Selective forgetting, or failure to mention important persons or life activities, may indicate denial or conflict.

□ THE AGGRESSIVE PSEUDO-INDEPENDENT PATIENT

An aggressive person is frequently restless and overactive. The patient may minimize or deny symptoms and try to take control of the situation (e.g., by directing you where to sit or indicating impatience or obvious displeasure). The patient may become angry when feeling control of the situation is in jeopardy. These outbursts frequently reflect the patient's anxiety. Try to acknowledge the anxiety. You may also help the patient regain control by moving away from the subject that provoked the anxiety. Indicating that the patient is helping may re-establish a much-needed sense of self-esteem. However, if, after all your efforts, the patient remains unwilling, the subject should be dropped, and you should move on to a subject that is neutral or conducive to bolstering the patient's self-esteem.

□ THE DEMANDING, DEPENDENT PATIENT

Demanding, dependent patients view themselves as deprived and neglected. They try to force others to take care of them (e.g., to adjust the bed, to lower the shades, etc). Such patients, feeling unmet needs, may become irritable and uncooperative.

□ THE PARANOID PATIENT

Paranoid patients are characterized by qualities of suspicion and accusation. The patient may ask, "Why do you want to know that?" "Who told you to ask me about that?" These questions are usually delusional and beyond an appeal to reason. Do not dispute the patient's false ideas; rather abandon the line of questioning that aroused the patient's suspicions. Occasionally such patients are dangerous, and become physically or verbally belligerent. Always remain close to the door. If you feel threatened in any way, trust your intuition and leave, reporting your concern to someone responsible for the patient's care.

□ THE DEPRESSED PATIENT

Depression of some degree accompanies every severe illness. It represents a response to loss (e.g., self-esteem, independence, sense of wholeness). Most persons quickly adapt to their illness and reassert their independence as soon as their medical condition is defined and stabilized.

When depression in a patient is more pervasive as a result of major illness from which full recovery is not expected or as a manifestation of a life-long personality pattern, then feelings of worthlessness, hopelessness, apathy, guilt, and loneliness are present. Depression may be manifested by tone of voice, posture, and speech. A severely depressed patient volunteers little and responds to questions with brief, relatively uninformative answers.

A statement like "You look sad," or "You look depressed," gives the patient an opportunity to talk about feelings. You need to be more active in interviewing a depressed person than other types of patients. Some depressed people have learned to be helpless (Seligman, 1975) and cling to others (including their health care providers) rather than assume responsibility for themselves. Helplessness is a way of life, and you may feel that patients put the burden of their lives, including getting well, on you. Ask direct questions earlier in the interview than you would with a more communicative patient. When this type of patient is helpful, express your appreciation as a way of countering the sense of helplessness. Suicidal thoughts should be asked about directly. Patients with such thoughts are often relieved that someone recognizes the seriousness of their condition.

☐ THE SEDUCTIVE PATIENT

Some patients may look for more than a professional doctor-patient relationship and develop romantic fantasies. Seductive behavior rarely emerges in an open, undisguised way. Sometimes the first indication of a potentially seductive situation is discovering in yourself romantic or sexual feelings about the patient. Don't feel ashamed or embarrassed and don't keep these things to yourself. Should such a situation develop, seek out someone you respect and discuss the problem. If not correctly handled, these situations can cause both you and the patient great harm. You may unconsciously encourage a seductive response by promising unrealistic expectations regarding the outcome of care. Don't become overly supportive or reassuring in an attempt to create trust and confidence. Telling your personal troubles to the patient is another kind of seductive behavior to be avoided.

If a patient is openly seductive, clarify the limits of the professional relationship without scolding or moralizing. You should also take the precaution of having a clinical assistant with you whenever you examine the patient, since sometimes seductive patients make false charges of unprofessional behavior against clinicians who do not comply with their sexual fantasies.

☐ THE "NOT DIFFICULT" PATIENT

Coming at the end of this long chapter on difficult relationships, a few words about the *not difficult* relationship are appropriate to restore balance. As health care professionals we spend so much time with sickness that we risk losing sight of health. Most people get along well without our help, or need it only occasionally. They have very adequate coping mechanisms to handle the medical and psychological stresses of life. The kinds of "difficult patients" described in this chapter are a small part of daily practice—although an important part. Don't get overwhelmed with their problems, however, and don't neglect to take notice and enjoy your healthy patients.

Healthy patients do more than contribute to the pleasure of practice—they provide an indispensable baseline against which to recognize disease. When in medical school I once asked our cardiology professor "How can I learn to recognize all these murmurs?" His reply was, "Listen to a thousand normal hearts." The more healthy people you interview and examine, the more acute will be your ability to recognize when people are ill.

Seeing a healthy patient offers an opportunity for health promotion. Sometimes the oppotunities to promote health are not obvious. A high school student who needs an "OK for football," for example, can be in and out of your office in five minutes, but taking extra time can open up discussions about sexual concerns, identity, relationships at home, alcohol, street drugs, and career planning. You have to take the first step. "Just another routine physical" can become a uniquely valuable opportunity to promote the health of the healthy.

□ A Strength Diagnosis

A balanced view of difficult patients recognizes not only their predominant problems or personality characteristics but also their strengths. Martens (1986) tells of a middle-aged man who was dying of metastatic cancer. His clinical problems included painful mouth lesions and poor nutrition resulting from chemotherapy, marked fatigue, financial problems, and the anxiety of approaching death. But the patient was also strongly motivated to maintain his independence, had a strong family support system, and had a will to live that sustained him through many of the stresses of therapy. Martens recommends that a "strength" diagnosis be made based on a patient's positive resources ". . . from which he can draw emotional or physical energy or an established lifestyle that fosters wellness."

□ Creating a Positive Response

Although this chapter has focused on patients "who most physicians would dread to treat," it would be a serious omission not to emphasize that the same processes that create a negative clinical atmosphere can also generate a positive one. Thus, greeting people in a smiling, cheerful way generates a similar response from others. You can "define a situation" in either a positive or negative way by the attitude you take. A person who may be regarded as "hostile" may live in a harsh world where everyone else is (or appears to be) hostile. Your ability to respond in unexpectedly positive ways may turn a difficult situation around. You can literally create for an embattled patient a small refuge of caring and kindness, which may initiate wholesome changes whose influence goes far beyond your brief time with the patient.

☐ REFERENCES AND READINGS

Anderson RO: The physician as an enabler of the chemically dependent patient. Postgrad Med 1986; 79:207–214.

Barsky AJ: Patients who amplify bodily sensations. Ann Intern Med 1979; 91:63–70.

Barsky AJ, Klerman GL: Overview: Bodily complaints and somatic styles. Am J Psychiatry 1983; 140:273–283.

Dewald PA: Counter-transference. In: Psychotherapy, New York, Basic Books, 1964, Chap 15.

Dewald PA: Transference. In: Psychotherapy, New York, Basic Books, 1964, Chap 12.

Dimsdale JE: Delays and slips in medical diagnosis. Perspect Biol Med 1984; 27:213–220.

Gorlin R, Zucker HD: Physicians' reaction to patients. New Engl J Med 1983; 308:1059–1063.

Hodle SF: What doctors dislike most about patients. Physicians' Management 1984; Nov:267–277.

Groves JE: Taking care of the hateful patient. N Engl J Med 1978; 298:883–887.

Klein D, Najman J. Kohrman AF, et al: Patient characteristics that elicit negative responses from family physicians. J Fam Pract 1982; 14:881–888.

Martens K: Let's diagnose strengths, not just problems. Am J Nurs 1986; 86:192–193.

Reiser DE, Schroder AK: After the interview. In: Patient Interviewing: The Human Dimension. Baltimore, Williams & Wilkins, 1980, Chap 7.

Seligman MEP: Helplessness. San Francisco, W H Freeman, 1975.

Smith RC: Teaching interviewing skills to medical students: The issue of countertransference. J Med Educ 1984; 59:582–588.

CHAPTER 21

THE FAMILY INTERVIEW

Gerri S. Lamb, M.S., R.N. *
Certified Adult Nurse Practitioner

When caring for patients, you often come in contact with members of their families. Even if family members are not present during the interview, their influence is considerable. Before you see the patient, the family often has been involved in interpreting and treating the symptoms and in deciding whether professional help is needed. After your visit, the family may play a decisive role in whether treatment plans are followed. Families have a significant effect on how individuals take care of themselves—or don't take care of themselves.

Interviewing family members and attending to information about the patient's family has several benefits:

1. Rapport with the patient's family enlists their positive contributions to the patient's treatment plan.

2. Information about the family may suggest possible causes or contributors to the patient's present symptoms.

3. Knowledge of the family environment in which the patient carries on his daily life activities contributes to more realistic treatment plans.

There is no universal format for interviewing or collecting information about families. As in other areas of the interview, become familiar with key categories of information and then experiment with different interviewing techniques. What follows are some suggestions for a systematic approach to collecting family data as you interview patients, either in the context of a limited Problem-Centered interview or a more comprehensive Health Promotion evaluation. Overt family pathology, such as domestic violence, sexual or

---

*At the time this chapter was written: Assistant Professor, College of Nursing, University of Arizona. Currently a doctoral candidate at the University of Arizona.

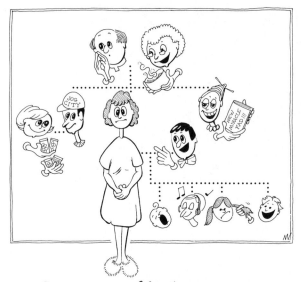

The influence of family members is
considerable.

physical abuse, or severe emotional or physical deprivation will not be discussed other than to indicate that such problems exist and need specialized professional help.

Thinking about families is different than thinking about individuals. A shifting of mental gears is needed to change your focus from one person to a set of people bonded by complex ties. Families are more than a sum of their individual members.

The family is experienced by each individual in a uniquely personal way. Don't be surprised if you hear differing accounts of the same situation from different family members. Ask for other family members' perspectives before drawing conclusions that may have significant impact on diagnoses and treatment plans. For example, an elderly man describes his middle-aged daughter as "detached and uncaring"; the daughter seems sincere in saying she loves her father but feels overwhelmed and unable to deal with the responsibilities of caring for an ill parent.

☐ Rationale and Content

You encounter family information during both a Health Promotion and a Problem-Centered interview. The patient's family is a focus of attention in the categories of Family Medical History and Personal/Social History. Obtaining useful information in these categories depends on understanding the rationale for each item of information gathered about the family.

Consider why you are asking for information about the patient's family.

Family data are part of Risk Factor assessment. Family events play a significant part in the development, continuation, and alleviation of a number of presenting symptoms. In a broader sense, questions about relationships in the family provide valuable data about the family's effectiveness in carrying out multiple functions that are closely related to the health of its members. Families have a major reponsibility for fostering healthy behaviors and for providing an environment in which each of its members is cared for physically and emotionally. Clearly, families differ in their abilities to carry out each of their functions. With this in mind, screening questions provide clues about how well the family is doing and if it needs help.

Information about the family is often divided into two major categories—function and structure. *Function* includes each of the activities that the family is responsible for carrying out, i.e., the protection of family members' health, socialization of children. *Structure* refers to the number of family members available to act as resources and the way families organize themselves to carry out each of their functions. Structure includes patterns that the family has developed for communication, decision making, distribution of power, and sharing of feelings. Effective (healthy) families have many of the following characteristics: (1) members communicate clearly and directly, (2) members solve problems together, (3) decision-making responsibilities are shared, (4) family members share a sense of cohesiveness, yet respect each person's "differences," and (5) parents work together to meet the needs of their children. No single characteristic distinguishes between a well functioning and a dysfunctional family. Rather, systematic attention to clusters of characteristics alerts you to problem areas or strengths.

□ Health Promotion

Information obtained from the Family History and Personal/Social History provides a baseline picture of the family, including components of structure and function.

Family Health History focuses on the occurrence of hereditary and contagious disease and also provides information about family structure—who's in the family; who's missing owing to divorce, death, or desertion. The presence of illness in the family may provide clues about possible sources of stress that members deal with on a day-to-day basis: a child with leukemia, a parent with Alzheimer's disease, alcoholism in several members. These risk factors may influence the patient's ability to care for himself or to follow your recommendations. The impact of the family illness on the patient can be ascertained without losing the flow of the interview; you can ask, "How has that been for you?" "What kinds of changes has that made in your life?" If the response indicates a need to pursue the topic, acknowledge the patient's feelings and indicate that you will return to the subject later during the present visit or at a future time.

Personal/Social History includes relevant family and social information, daily activities, and health habits, with an emphasis on those factors that contribute to an overall evaluation of the patient's health. Initial questions are open-ended with the purpose of getting a broad picture of family life, for example, "How are things going at home?" "How are your children doing?" "How are you getting along with your parents?" Patient responses will guide whether further discussion is indicated. Pay attention to nonverbal communication or unclear communications such as "OK. . .I guess," or "As well as can be expected."

Consider how to respond to honest and sometimes troubled replies, e.g., "I'm not getting along with my wife," "Having a child is not what I expected." While you may not be prepared to pursue such comments in detail, acknowledge that family matters may be as much a source of pain as the presenting physical symptoms. Also, consider the influence of the family in the development and maintenance of healthy behaviors (regular dental care, balanced meals, use of seat belts) as well as its impact on detrimental habits. A general question such as "What kinds of things do you do to keep your family healthy?" often yields useful information.

Detailed questions about family structure and function are not usually included in the first interview unless responses to open-ended questions indicate that there is an immediate problem that needs to be discussed. Questions about daily activities, relaxation, and recreation provide general information about the amount of time spent with family members and types of joint activities. Remember: weekend activities may differ from a description of the "typical day."

Final questions that are used to close the initial interview, like "What does your chest pain mean to you?" may be expanded to include ideas of other family members, e.g., "What does your wife think about your chest pain?" Sometimes it may be easier for the patient to attribute his or her own concerns to another family member. Response to this question provides additional clues about family function, e.g., "I didn't tell my wife about my chest pain."

A brief questionnaire, such as the Family APGAR (Smilkstein, 1978), is another means of collecting general information about family function during initial assessment. The Family APGAR allows family members to rate their satisfaction with different aspects of their family life, such as expressions of affection, emotional support at times of trouble, time spent together, and participation in problem solving; these are good starting points for discussion and are useful in tracking changes over time. More detailed family assessment instruments are also available; references to some of these are at the conclusion of this chapter.

☐ Comprehensive Family Information

Watch for clues suggesting that more detailed family information is needed to gain a clearer perspective on the patient's problem and for developing an effective treatment program. For example, does the patient become more anxious during discussion of family matters? do certain family topics appear over and over? are some family members never mentioned? are there inconsistencies in the patient's verbal and nonverbal communication when talking about family members?

The following are situations in which gathering more detailed family information is indicated:

The patient has symptoms that he or she believes are related to what's going on in the family.

A middle-aged woman seeks care for fatigue and difficulty sleeping, which she relates to the unexplained departure of her husband of 25 years.

The patient or a group of family members come to you for assistance in dealing with a problem behavior in some other member of the family.

A middle-aged son brings in his mother who insists on living alone despite his protests. He wants your help in considering alternative living arrangements.

A parent wants to know how to respond to her three-year-old son's temper tantrums.

The patient's family is going through, or anticipating going through, a life cycle change involving predictable stress.

A young couple bring in their four-week-old son for his first well-child check.

A single parent comes in for her health maintenance visit and comments that her youngest child, who is 18, will be leaving for college in a few months.

The patient shows no improvement despite treatment.

After several weeks of diet counseling, an overweight woman with poorly controlled diabetes, shares, "My husband likes me fat and says he'll leave me if I lose weight."

The success of the treatment plan depends on active participation of family members.

A young boy is readmitted to the hospital in an acute asthmatic attack. His return home depends on his family's willingness and ability to modify the home environment and to provide continuing encouragement.

□ Interviewing Techniques

Interviewing techniques when dealing with family-related issues are those described in *Unit IV: Communication Techniques.* Transitional statements that focus the patient's attention to the social aspects of the family are sometimes needed to explain your reasons for asking about potentially sensitive family issues.

"We've talked in the past about how things are going at home for you. Sometimes, family problems can lead to headaches, chest pain. . ."

"I'd like to talk more about your family now."

"Many parents find that having a new baby creates a lot of changes for them. How has it been for you?"

Use of neutral terms like "change" or "adjustment" allows the patient to incorporate his own feelings about the positive or negative nature of the family event.

After asking open-ended questions about family life, select a few areas of family structure and function that will allow you to get a picture of how the family is working. Start with questions that are comfortable for you and that you feel will be acceptable to the patient.

The following are examples of categories of family information and sample questions.

Life Cycle/Development

"Families go through a lot of changes together—births, kids leaving home, parents growing older. What kinds of changes are going on in your family?"

"What kinds of changes are you expecting in the next few months/years? How well prepared do you feel your family is/will be for dealing with these changes?"

Communication

"How do people talk to each other in your family?"

"Are there special times to sit down and talk?"

"When you talk do you feel listened to?"

"Are all subjects all right to talk about, or are there some that are off limits?"

"Do people usually understand what you're trying to tell them?"

"How do you know when (Family Member) is happy, angry? How does (Family Member) know when you're happy, sad. . .? How do you let (Family Member) know when you need something from him?"

Decision-making/Power

"How are decisions made in your family?"

"Are family members able to work out problems together?"

"Who makes the rules? What happens when someone breaks a family rule?"

"Who wins arguments? Who has the last say?"

Feelings/Cohesiveness

"What do you like about the people in your family? What don't you like?"

"Do members of your family spend time together? Do they seem to enjoy these times?"

"How does it feel to be a member of your family?"

"How do people care about each other in your family?'

Dealing with Differentness

"How are members of your family like each other? How are they different?"

"How do people react when someone says or does something different? Is it okay to be different in your family?"

Supports/Resources

"Who/where do you go when you need some help?"

"What community organizations do you belong to?"

Family Goals

"If you could change one thing about your family, what would it be? What would you keep the same?"

□ Observing Families

Watching families in action in the medical office or during a home visit is an effective means of collecting family data. Families, like individuals, provide a wealth of information through verbal and nonverbal messages. Observation can provide initial impressions about family relationships, communication, decision-making, discipline, and sharing of affection. Initial impressions provide hypotheses about family functioning; you will need to validate these hypotheses during subsequent interactions and discussion with family members. Nonverbal communication, such as seating arrangements, may provide clues about family structure, e.g., does the husband/father sit three chairs away from his wife and child who are sitting very close to each other? Do family members look at each other when they talk? Do they touch each other? Who talks to whom? Are there some people who rarely talk? Do members of this family speak for themselves? Do people talk for each other? How do parents respond to a child who is frightened, angry, emptying the drawers of your examining table?

And one final observation: how do *you* feel when you're with this family—comfortable, angry, threatened, depressed. . . ? Your response will give you a sense of how family members are feeling and what it may be like to be a member of this family.

□ Involving the Family

Interviewing techniques discussed in *Unit V: Interview Procedures*, are useful in working with families as well as individuals. Establishing rappport with family members is as important as it is with an individual. Additions to good interviewing style discussed earlier include:

Introduce yourself to each family member who is present during the interview.

Establish eye contact briefly with each person as you introduce yourself.

Request the patient's opinion about the amount of family participation desired.

"Did you want (family member) to stay for this part of our discussion?"

Provide a brief explanation if you prefer to interview the patient without family members present.

Respond in appropriate depth to concerns of family members.

Request permission to discuss topics that have been shared with you in private prior to bringing them up in the presence of other family members. Earlier comments about confidentiality also apply to families.

Request permission to discuss topics that have been shared with you during the session with other professionals as necessary.

□ REFERENCES AND READINGS

Epstein N, Baldwin L, Bishop D: The McMaster family assessment device. Journal of Marital and Family Therapy 1983;9:171–180.
Juberg RC: Making the family history relevant. JAMA 1972;220:122–123.
Lewis JM, Beavers WR, Gossett JT, et al: No Single Thread; Psychological Health in Family Systems. New York, Brunner/Mazel, 1976.

Pless I, Satterwaite B: A measure of family functioning and its application. Social Science and Medicine 1973;7:613–621.

Pratt L: Family Structure and Effective Health Behavior. Boston, Houghton Mifflin, 1976.

Resnikof F: Ten key questions for understanding the family as patient. Journal of Marital and Family Therapy 1981;7:135–142.

Satir V: Peoplemaking. Palo Alto, Science and Behavior Books, 1972.

Sedgwick R, Hildebrand S: Family health assessment. Nurse Practitioner 1981;6:37–45.

Smilkstein G: The Family APGAR: A proposal for a family function test and its use by physicians. J Fam Pract 1978;6:1231–1239.

Thrower S: The family circle method for integrating family systems concepts in family medicine. J Fam Pract 1982;15:451–457.

CHAPTER 22

PEDIATRIC INTERVIEWING

Ronald Fischler, M.D. *

When your patient is a child, your approach to the interview differs from that used when interviewing adults. Much or all the history is obtained from a parent.† Young children lack the language skills needed for a detailed description of their illness, nor do they know about their past history. Older children, of course, are able to provide you with useful information that supplements the parent's history. Stages of a child's development are a major determinant of the pediatric interview. Caring for a one-month-old infant is a lot different than caring for a nine-year-old child; you'll need different interviewing styles for different age groups. Often you are really dealing with two patients, the child and the parent. The parent, the child's "agent," has needs that influence, sometimes to an important degree, the direction and kind of care given.

Illnesses, both minor and major, in young children frequently are atypical. Potentially serious diseases such as meningitis or appendicitis are deceptive, especially early in their course, and the diagnosis may be missed or delayed. Minor diseases, especially some viral illnesses, provoke truly frightening, although usually harmless, manifestations such as convulsions or scary temper-

---

*Director, Pediatric Ambulatory Care Center, St. Joseph's Hospital, Phoenix, Arizona
†The term "parent" is used for editorial simplicity, but refers, in real life, to "caretakers": father, mother, grandparents, foster parents, relatives, or even neighbors.

ature elevations. Abuse and neglect are usually accompanied by deliberate deception and are presented to you as some kind of accident or unexplained illness. And chronic illnesses may appear as a confusing blend of acute conditions and abnormalities of growth and development. In all these instances, your ability to gather accurate information and to maintain rapport with both child and parent are the foundations of effective care. Success depends on being a astute listener and a sensitive observer.

□ Student Roles and Concerns

There is a refreshing quality associated with caring for children, and most students feel at ease after some initial anxiety. Even children with potentially fatal diseases or chronic handicaps will, if given a chance, welcome you into their lives. To qualify, you need only to be honest with children and to have an accepting attitude. These qualities apply to your interactions with the child's parents, although in some situations, such as child abuse and neglect, cultivating a positive relationship is not easy.

□ Seeking Medical Care

Parents are the persons who seek care for their children. Usually the need is obvious. Sometimes, however, the reason for the visit is not clear, and you must look beneath the surface for the hidden agenda. Sometimes a parent, experiencing guilt about some issue unrelated to the child, anticipates punishment in the form of a fatal illness like leukemia befalling the child. Lack of basic health knowledge about children, especially with a first child, results in anxiety about minor symptoms. A parent's description of the child's health that is inconsistent with what you see—for example, an obviously healthy child being described as "always sick"—is a signal to explore below the surface.

□ Rapport

The same personal and professional qualities and communication skills needed to establish rapport with adults apply to children. In some ways the task of establishing rapport with children is easier. Your youthful appearance, for example, will be an asset. Casual dress is acceptable; in fact, if a young child has had unpleasant past experiences with the medical profession, anything *except* a white coat will be appropriate.

Active listening and constant alertness for a "hidden agenda" are particularly important, since much of what you need to know must be inferred rather than learned from direct statements.

Honesty is paramount. Children sense dishonesty no matter how cleverly it is disguised. A false statement that "this won't hurt" will destroy trust, not only in your future relations, but possibly in the child's relations with other clinicians as well. Children learn the truth despite the strategies of adults to obscure it.

A 13-year-old girl with leukemia was seen regularly in the Pediatric Clinic. The family insisted that the child not be told the nature of her illness and the likelihood of its fatal outcome.

Her condition finally required hospitalization. The physician interviewing her on admission tactfully explored her understanding of her disease. She said very matter-of-factly that she though it must be something serious, and she believed she was going to die. Her reason: "Before I got sick my parents never went to church—now they go all the time."

☐ The *Fundamental Four*

The pediatric history is structured within the same *Fundamental Four* as used with the adult interview. The Present Illness focuses on the broad overview, plus symptom analysis using the *Sacred Seven*. Risk factor history for children is the same as with adults except for somewhat different content and emphasis.

The Past Medical History includes information on the mother's prenatal history and general health, the course of labor and delivery, and the neonatal course. Illnesses, accidents, and hospitalizations, the patient's immunization status and nutrition and physical growth are important too.

Family Medical History includes birth defects, hereditary conditions, and infant deaths.

Personal/Social History includes the child's development and behavior during infancy, early childhood, late childhood and adolescence. The composition of the household and a history of recent life stresses should also be obtained.

As with other histories, just how you classify a particular data element is somewhat arbitrary. Many pediatricians, for example, include Development and Behavior as part of the child's Past Medical History. The details of classification are not important as long as you understand the importance, in terms of diagnosis and treatment, of the information you obtain.

☐ The Problem-Centered Interview

Problem-centered care involves four major kinds of problems:
1. Minor acute illness.
2. Life-threatening acute illness.
3. Abuse and neglect.
4. Chronic illness.

These illnesses, especially in young children, frequently are atypical in their symptoms and signs, and not always easy to identify.

The *Sacred Seven* and the *Fundamental Four* provide structure for the history.

□ Health Promotion

□ WELL CHILD CARE

Building a relationship with the parents is a key element in well child care. (As a student this is difficult because frequent changes in clerkships prevent continuity of care and the establishment of a long-term relationship.)

Creating a tone of acceptance that helps the parent feel comfortable bringing up any concern is extremely important. Avoid setting yourself up as an authority who has all the answers; such an attitude puts the parent in the role of the passive recipient and creates dependence and insecurity rather than independence and confidence.

Having a checklist to guide you efficiently through the history, while allowing flexibility to deal with whatever concerns the parent is another key to success in well child care.

As society changes, so does the prevention and early detection focus of a Health Promotion Visit. Depression, suicide, automobile accidents, and substance abuse are, unfortunately, significant problems in the pediatric age group. Social adjustment at home and in school should always be evaluated.

A first visit for a Health Promotion assessment takes approximately 40–60 minutes. It begins with the Present Illness, essentially an assessment of the child's overall functioning. The Review of Systems is useful for this purpose. Then a comprehensive Past Medical History, Family Medical History, and Personal/Social History are compiled and recorded. At subsequent visits, the comprehensive Pediatric Database thus compiled gives you a quick overview of the child's history.

□ Procedure Basics

With younger children, especially, maintain the parent-child dyad: let the child sit on the parent's lap during the interview. Look at both when asking questions even though the child is too young for verbal understanding. To separate unnecessarily the parent and child is traumatic, creating fear and making your task more difficult.

Infants up to seven to nine months generally are not bothered by your presence as a "stranger"; however, after 7 to 9 months through 24 to 36 months strangers are perceived as frightening. Children of this age should be examined on their parent's lap. During the interview, cautiously approach the child by offering toys in a playful way, while making little eye contact at first until the child becomes comfortable. Allowing the child to first hold the tongue blade, flashlight, or stethoscope, and showing how you use them by demonstrating on the parent or a doll helps allay anxiety. Watch how a seasoned clinician uses these and other techniques to gently initiate the interview and examination. Making a game of the examination goes a long way towards gaining cooperation.

Touching during the examination is a primary means of communication with infants. Even when restraining is needed, it can be done in a firm but gentle way that expresses your concern. Also, a pleasant manner and the ability to laugh will have your pediatric patients laughing and smiling with you.

With older children and adolescents, gaining participation is important. Initiate the conversation around some area of interest to the child—sports, book or TV characters, school, or work. Once rapport is established, the patient's concerns and level of understanding of health or illness can be addressed. With adolescents, some or all of the interview and examination should be without the presence of the parents. This acknowledges the fact that the child is nearly grown-up and responsible.

☐ Interviewing in the Hospital

Children in the hospital generally have serious, acute illnesses or worsening of a chronic illness. They may have been admitted because outpatient treatment has failed, or because attempts to make a specific diagnosis have been unsuccessful. They may be critically ill and in an intensive care unit, and are likely to be quite different than their usual selves. Their parents may be anxious and worried, sometimes even hysterical. If the child's condition is unstable, the interview is limited to a Problem-Centered history until the child is stabilized. An efficient use of staff energy is to have one member of the health care team interview the parents in a quiet room while others care for the child. This technique has the benefit of calming the parents so that a more complete database can be obtained, while at the same time insuring that the child is appropriately treated.

☐ Interviewing in the Medical Office

Most office visits involve a Problem-Centered interview. The typical outpatient visit is a 15 to 20 minute encounter for well children and for those with acute illnesses. Therefore, outpatient interviewing must be brief, problem-centered, focused, and efficient. Efficient does not mean rushed. The key to the brief interview is *relevance*. The Present Illness is detailed, followed by relevant questions related to the risk factors. Going through the mind of the clinician are questions such as: Is the problem serious? Urgent? Can it be managed in the office today or is more time needed? Does the child need to be hospitalized?

□ Difficult Interviewing Situations

□ THE ANXIOUS PARENT

There is often a degree of anxiety connected with all visits of a doctor. Sometimes this is obvious, at other times it is not; instead, the child's symptoms, as presented by the parent, seem out of proportion to the child's appearance. In particular, pay attention to how you feel at the end of the interview. With anxious parents there is often a lack of closure—a sense of "unfinished business." The parent seems unsatisfied although the reasons may be obscure. When you feel this way, it is helpful to say, "I get the feeling that you are still worried, or that something else we haven't discussed is concerning you." This will often flush out hidden agendas for discussion at that time, or some future visit. It may also signal the need for professional counseling.

□ THE HANDICAPPED OR CHRONICALLY ILL CHILD

Encountering a child with a major handicap can be an uncomfortable experience. You may feel a sense of revulsion by the child's appearance or behavior. Pity for the parent, and fear for yourself should you someday have a child with a similar condition, are common reactions. These feelings can get in the way of your objectivity unless you acknowledge them and develop strategies to cope with them.

There are four issues in caring for a child with a chronic illness or handicap:
1. The medical condition and how it is managed.
2. The child's psychological and social adjustment: the child's limitations but also the child's strengths.
3. The family's adjustment in terms of emotional and financial demands, including social support from family, friends, and community organizations.
4. Education issues: encouragement of child and family to take full advantage of educational opportunities.

Parents of seriously handicapped children characteristically experience a normal grief reaction after learning the diagnosis. The grief process, which may last for months or years, involves these stages:
1. Shock.
2. Denial and disbelief.
3. Anger.
4. Bargaining.
5. Guilt.
6. Acceptance.

Acceptance implies a good understanding of the condition, and a knowledge of its cause (if known) and treatment. Early in the grieving process, parents may be depressed, and focus on what their child *cannot* do. When they accept the child's condition, they are generally pleased to report all of the things their child *can do*; there is also ample time for themselves as individuals and for other siblings, and they appear happy and content. It is easy to underestimate the emotional resources of a family dealing with a situation that at first seems overwhelming. Pity, overprotectiveness, or offering unrealistic hopes are some possible responses; none of these will help the situation or your relationship with the patient. In summary, the interview of the handicapped or chronically ill child involves seeing the illness in the context of the child's and family's ability to function.

□ THE ABUSED OR NEGLECTED CHILD

Evaluating a child who may be the victim of abuse or neglect is among the most difficult of all pediatric interviews. You may find yourself angry at the parent suspected of abuse, uncertain of your legal obligations, and anxious about confronting abusing parents and incurring their anger.

The key to the diagnosis of abuse or neglect is a high index of suspicion about illnesses or injuries that are inadequately explained during the interview. Active listening for inconsistencies or the reporting of improbable events helps you to judge whether of not abuse occurred. Open-ended questions such as "Tell me what happened," which require the parent to construct the events leading up to the child's injury, may leave you feeling their report is a fabrication. Injuries involving the face, buttocks, thighs, or genitals are especially suspect. Inappropriate delays in seeking medical treatment, for example, injuries or acute illnesses that are several days old, are also suspicious of a lack of appropriate parenting.

The child's general appearance often supports an impression of abuse or neglect: the child may be dirty or uncared for, may show below normal growth (weight more depressed than height for no obvious reason), or may be unusually quiet. Developmental delays, poor social interaction, inappropriate or unrealistic expectations by parents for their child, such as expecting the child to be toilet trained during the first months of life, are also valuable clues, as are parents' characterization of their child as "bad" or "difficult."

Coping with the doctor-parent interaction in child abuse cases is helped by the awareness that parents usually care about their child even though they have abused him or her. Abusing parents usually want help even if they do not ask for help directly. Child Protective Services and laws designed to protect children usually result in restoration of family functioning; only rarely are children permanently separated from their families. However, during the initial investigation process, families often perceive the investigation as intrusive and threatening, and they often feel accused by everyone. It is helpful to be sympathetic with what the parents are experiencing and convey the message that while your first obligation is the welfare of their child, you are also concerned about them. Explain that the laws require you to ask these questions and report to Child Protective Services, but that you will keep them informed, will stand by them, and will provide help at any time.

□ ALTERNATIVE LIFESTYLES

You will occasionally encounter parents whose lifestyles, attitudes, or beliefs concerning child care differ markedly from the norm. For example, they may prefer raw goat's milk, with its risk of gastrointestinal infection or tuberculosis, to commercial formula, or decline immunizations for their children. Your initial reaction to such parents may be one of "righteous indignation," which will interfere with establishing rapport. Generally such parents are concerned and take good care of their children and want only to participate actively in decisions concerning their children's health care. If they are accepted on this basis, they will listen to your information and advice. If given appropriate time to make a decision they will often compomise and, for example, allow tetanus and polio immunizations and switch to nutritionally adequate and safe pasteurized goat's milk with supplemental vitamins. On the other hand, if you feel that a parent's beliefs and practices will cause the child significant harm, such as refusing chemotherapy for leukemia in favor of Laetrile, then Child Protective Services or a similar agency must be notified.

Giving information is one way to achieve your objectives while still allowing the parents to maintain their self-esteem, for example, saying, "The importance for this procedure isn't always understood—let me explain why it is so important for your child." Establishing a common bond with parents by "Doing what is best for your child" is often the basis for overcoming initial resistance.

□ Identifying with the Child

Physicians who care for children usually like children. It is possible, however, to like children too much and to lose objectivity in the process. We as adults retain something of our own childhood. If it wasn't a happy one, it is possible to see ourselves in our patient (the mistaken identity process discussed in *Chapter 20: Difficult Relationships*), setting the stage for identification and inappropriate emotional involvement with the child. Such involvement may extend beyond the child and lead to an adversarial relationship with the parents or with community agencies involved in the child's welfare.

□ A Final Thought

Caring for children is a challenge—it can also be a source of great satisfaction. Children are resilient, often considerably more so than adults. Even children with severe chronic disabling or fatal conditions seem to cope remarkably well in spite of our inability to cure them. A potential hazard for us as physicians (since we know the adverse medical possibilities) is to become enslaved in our fears and uncertainties. We may come to see children as fragile, vulnerable, and dependent on our perfect knowledge and experitise, thus communicating our sense of worry to the parents. There is another way to cope. Rather than spend needless energy worrying about all the possible adverse outcomes, invest your efforts in a positive, common-sense approach. Provide health information to support the parent's ability to be a good caretaker: to take reasonable precautions to prevent illness, to promote health and safety, and to ask for help when needed. For all of its serious aspects, parenting should also be fun and educational, and as physicians, we can help make it so.

□ REFERENCES AND READINGS

Council on Scientific Affairs: AMA diagnostic and treatment guidelines concerning child abuse and neglect. JAMA 1985; 254:796–800.
Fulginiti VA: Pediatric Clinical Problem Solving. Baltimore, Williams & Wilkins, 1981.
Korsch BM, Negrete V: Doctor-patient communication. Sci Am 1972;227:66–74.

CHAPTER

23

INTERVIEWING THE OLDER PATIENT

Marlene Bluestein, M.D. *

Interviewing older persons is both challenging and rewarding. It is challenging because of the spectrum and complexity of their medical and psychosocial conditions; rewarding because of the difference you can make in their quality of life and their overall health status. Geriatrics is a rapidly growing medical speciality, and as the population ages, the demand for health services by persons in the older age groups is accelerating. Medicare and other forms of health insurance now translate the needs of seniors into the ability to obtain quality care.

As in every sphere of clinical practice, the interview and the health history are the foundation of rapport, diagnosis, and therapy. The physical examination has its place, of course, but the atypical nature of many physical findings in the older person places increased reliance on knowing what to suspect and look for, based on the history, when beginning the physical examination.

☐ Student Roles and Attitudes

Older patients, as a rule, welcome students. Often these patients hunger for a sympathetic listener. You will have the opportunity to share in a lifetime of experiences of persons who have succeeded, or failed, in every aspect of life. The chance to learn and benefit from their experiences is a unique opportunity if you choose to accept it.

Aversion to older patients is not uncommon among clinicians. The inter-

---

*Assistant Professor, Department of Internal Medicine, University of Arizona College of Medicine, Tucson, Arizona. Chief of Geriatric Medicine, Tucson Veterans Administration Hospital

view takes longer, and the patient may not be able to give as detailed a history as younger persons. You may displace onto a patient your feelings about your parents. Physicians may see in the elderly their own aging.

Older persons frustrate physicians in other ways. The complexity of geriatric problems and the co-existence of medical and psychosocial problems require a complicated and sometimes contradictory set of treatment plans. Illnesses of older persons rarely are as described in medical school lectures or in textbooks; some conditions are not well understood, and others appear in atypical ways. A relatively simple condition like appendicitis in a 75-year-old person, for example, is easily misdiagnosed even by an experienced physician. Finally, many conditions of the elderly are not curable, and the fact that older persons die more often than younger persons counters some clinicians need for success and mastery.

These considerations suggest the need to redefine one's philosophy about what to expect when caring for older persons. An unknown physician once summarized realistic expectations as:

To cure sometimes. To relieve often. To comfort always.

In this context, caring for older persons can be as medically challenging and personally satisfying as any other type of practice.

□ Seeking Medical Care

Older patients see their physicians for the same general reasons as do younger persons: to relieve discomfort and maintain optimal health. This general statement requires modifications in the context of geriatric medicine. Chronic disease predominantes, and acute illness may be attributed instead to some chronic condition. Expectations of older persons differ from those of younger ones. A certain amount of disability is expected as an inevitable part of aging. Indeed, some patients are resigned to live with conditions for which significant relief or cure is possible. Even small improvement in conditions such as arthritis is acceptable and appreciated.

In addition to medical care, the older patient will turn to you for help with nonmedical problems affecting everyday living. Frequently you and your staff are the patient's only resource in meeting all kinds of difficulties. Limited funds, loneliness, unsatisfactory living conditions, recreational needs, transportation, and other problems may be handed over to you for solutions.

Older patients have the same kind of hidden agendas and the same sick role behaviors as discussed in *Chapter 3: Seeking and Accepting Health Care.* And there are always surprises: one woman paid $120 for an examination she really did not need in order to ask me, at the end of the visit, "Do you know any nice older men who would like to meet a nice older woman like me?"

□ **Rapport**

When an older patient is ill, "my doctor" may be the most important person in his or her life. Anyone who is sick has lost power, and older persons keenly experience their vulnerability. And because they are so dependent on you, they cannot risk expressing resentment or dissatisfaction with the services you provide. You may be an unwitting part of a conspiracy of silence, which can be overcome only by a sensitivity to verbal and nonverbal communications, and a deliberate effort at open, honest communication.

Aspects of relating to older persons that have been shown to be especially helpful are discussed in the following paragraphs.

Respect their need to be independent. The less independence older persons have, the more they wish it. Tact is invaluable. For example, one physician, when facing the not infrequent situation of a patient refusing to go to the hospital despite obvious need, empowers the patient by saying, "I would feel better if you would go to the hospital—I would rest easier."

Providing opportunities to talk about their accomplishments, their families, and whatever else maintains and strengthens their self-esteem facilitates rapport. Asking about grandchildren is usually a winner (don't forget to ask if the patient has a picture). Many older men link much of their identity with their work and appreciate the chance to describe their past achievements.

Respect their "scientific understanding," even if it isn't very scientific. For example, a man with a multiplicity of problems explained everything on the basis of arthritis. While this violated modern knowledge (he had a rare sarcoma), what mattered was how much sense the diagnosis made in the context of his understanding of disease. If a patient thi 'ks you are wrong about what is the matter, cooperation with you in care is not likely. In the patient's culture nonphysicians may play a respected role. In the Southwest, for example, the Mexican-American *curanderos* provide very real benefits to patient care, and Indian Health Service physicians respect and make a place for the traditional *medicine man.* Scientific or not, folk culture is a helpful tool.

Give older persons a say in decisions made about their care. To varying degrees, all patients feel some loss of autonomy when dealing with the health care system. Some may not want to be involved, feeling that "You are the doctor." However, in asking you show respect for them as individuals. And when they do want to participate in decisions affecting them, not to involve them is a serious omission. They may feel more like objects than persons.

Avoid any public show of their deficits. Medical care is sometimes not as private as it should be. Examining a patient in a two-bed or four-bed hospital room may be embarrassing if the patient is unable to perform accurately simple mental status examination tests, and other patients overhear what is going on. Similarly, try to avoid any testing in which the patient becomes aware of failing. For example, in mental status testing, avoid saying, "Now I am going to ask you some simple questions." Not knowing the answers to some "simple" questions is distressing. Far better is to say, "Now I am going to ask you a series of questions—some are simple and some are not so simple."

Be cautious about expressing empathy. For a 25-year-old medical student to tell an 80-year-person, "I understand how you feel" may not be convincing. But sometimes saying, "My grandmother had something similar," or "I felt that way when I was in the hospital" does reduce the patient's sense of isolation.

Don't hesitate to admit that you are wrong and the patient is right. Recently, I placed a patient who had metastatic carcinoma on low-dose, around-the-clock narcotics, which is often a good way to control pain. This patient, however, became overly sedated, and told me with some anger that she didn't like feeling that way. She was a former nurse and knew what she was talking about. She was right and I was wrong, and I told her, "Yes, you are right. I thought regular shots would avoid making you sick to your stomach, and would be helpful, but I can see that the drowsiness and confusion they are causing aren't good for you." Admitting this strengthened, rather than weakened, our relationship. Patients often know better than you do what is best for them: seek their advice when appropriate.

Be constantly alert to covert calls for help. Many injustices befall the elderly who, nevertheless, feel they cannot risk complaining. Physical and mental abuse are more common than generally appreciated, yet the victim may actually defend the abuser rather than risk abandonment. The elderly are the target of fraudulent schemes and criminal activity, but even if the activity is discovered, the victim may be threatened into silence. Patients often send hidden messages, however, hoping you will come to their rescue. If you suspect an older patient is being victimized, consult a knowledgeable social worker or other appropriate professional.

Depression is a common but frequently missed condition because it appears in the guise of clinging and complaining about which you feel you can do little. If such behaviors are the surface manifestations of depression, you can do a great deal to relieve the underlying condition.

☐ Content of the Interview

As with other patients who come to see you because of a specific problem, focusing on the Present Illness, their current health functioning and a detailed description of their symptoms is what they expect and what is most useful. In addition to defining symptoms of illness as precisely as possible, you will want to assess the patient's activities of daily living, including the capability to bathe, dress, go to the toilet, prepare and eat food, maintain bowel and bladder control, move about, and manage basic financial affairs. The quality of sleep is important.

Past Medical History and Family Medical History, although helpful, may be of less value than in a younger person. For one thing, the patient's recall may be inaccurate and details may be lacking or unnecessary. If, for example, a patient says that her mother, father, two brothers, and a son all died of "heart attacks," this information is enough to suggest a "family history of heart disease," even if the patient does not recall the exact details. Also, keep in mind that conditions diagnosed decades ago may have relatively little validity in the context of current knowledge. Documenting a previous diagnosis by obtaining previous records is often necessary if the matter is essential. Information about current medications is particularly important—not only medications prescribed for the patient, but also those prescribed for the patient's friends and relatives, and taken on their recommendations. Often the easiest way to obtain information about medications is to ask the patient to bring in all the medicines being taken. Be sure to include over-the-counter drugs in your request.

The *Personal/Social History* will occupy much of your attention. As has already been mentioned, you and other health care providers occupy an important, sometimes dominant, role in many older persons' life concerns. While this does not mean that you need to become a social worker as well as a physician, knowing about the older person's psychosocial environment enables you to provide more effective care. Some Personal and Social data are worth emphasizing in your data base.

Social Support. Who is at home? Does the patient have family or close friends who would help at home (it is a good idea to get names and telephone numbers)? If your patient lives with someone else, what will happen if one partner dies? Don't overlook the role of pets as companions.

Occupation. "Retired from. . ." Many conditions like respiratory diseases have their beginnings in occupations such as mining decades ago.

Nutrition. The nutritional adequacy of the older person's diet is an important factor in the patient's overall health status and ability to recover from illness. A food diary maintained for a week or two is an excellent method to evaluate what the patient is eating. A home visit is another way to estimate how well the patient is eating.

Exercise. Even a simple walking program does wonders for an older person's physical and mental health. Swimming is excellent exercise because it makes gentle demands on the entire body, and has few physical risks that might cause injury. Of course, many older people participate in vigorous exercises such as tennis, golf, and dancing.

Neighborhood. Is the patient safe outside? Some elderly are literally trapped in their own homes or apartments, and live in continuous fear for their safety.

Finances. While many elderly persons have a very limited income, others have adequate resources. Tact is needed in discussing money to preserve the patient's self-esteem. Care should be taken to explain that your interest is not a personal one, but only that the patient should be able to afford necessary care.

Spiritual/Religious Resources. Personal beliefs have a major influence on a person's ability to live successfully. Also, religious organizations offer many social opportunities, provide support groups, and can help with tasks of daily living.

Sexual History. Don't underestimate the sexuality of the older person. Some have a vigorous, satisfying sex life and others experience severe frustrations. Many older persons are reluctant to discuss sexuality unless you encourage communication with questions like "Is sex an issue?" or "How can I help?"

Issues you may have to anticipate and take the lead in discussing include:

☐ Lack of arousal.
☐ Impotency.
☐ Sexual concerns associated with prostate difficulties.
☐ Opportunities for privacy for couples living in nursing homes.
☐ Appropriateness of masturbation.
☐ Incontinence, while not truly a sexual matter, may be considered by the patient as "too private" a matter to be discussed.

☐ Health Promotion or Preventive Medicine

Accidents and preventable illnesses deserve special attention in history-taking. Falls in the home are a leading cause of hospitalization. Many accidents can be avoided by simple measures such as installing grab bars in the bathroom and removing small rugs. A Visiting Nurse or a relative can easily address these matters, but it is your obligation to identify the risk during the history-taking process and to initiate remedial action. The immunization status of older patients, particularly regarding influenza and pneumonia, is a part of any comprehensive health assessment.

☐ Verbal Interview Techniques

Open-ended questions are valuable for getting the broad picture. I always start an interview by asking, "What is concerning you; tell me about it." If the reply is "*Everything* is bothering me," then I ask, "Tell me the three things that are bothering you the most." Not *every* patient can respond to open-ended questions, but it is always worth the try, and when it is successful you'll learn the patient's perspective of the problem. Some techniques that help in interviewing:

1. *Speak clearly*, not necessarily loudly. Sit so the patient can see you—a certain amount of reading lips and gesturing helps the patient who has a hearing loss.

2. *Be patient.* Older persons may be slow in recalling information (they have a lot to review before finding the answer). Avoid filling in the answers for the patient.

□ Nonverbal Communication

Anxiety often is expressed by a tremor or a need to urinate—watch for signs that a patient might like to interrupt the interview in order to void. Speech-impaired patients (such as those who have had strokes) may rely primarily on gestures to communicate.

□ Interview Procedure Basics

Help the patient remember your name; repeat it several times. A name tag helps if the lettering is large enough to be seen at a distance (most name tags are legible only to the wearer).

Watch the patient in action whenever possible. Escort your patient in from the waiting room rather than asking someone else to do it. Watching how a person gets up and moves about will tell you much about the patient's overall mobility and general health that you cannot learn in the examining room. If appropriate, watch how the patient dresses or undresses to get an idea of dexterity and ability to handle small objects.

Assess reliability early in the interview if you question the patient's ability to provide accurate information. A few screening questions measuring orientation and current knowledge tell if significant cognitive impairment is present (see *Chapter 16: Procedure Basics* for a simple mental status test). You may hesitate to ask questions which the patient might consider insulting, but this can be tactfully done without hurting the patient's feelings. For example, you might say, "Mrs. Smith, I have a feeling you are having some problem with your memory. I'd like to ask a few memory-type questions." Most of the time the patient seems almost relieved that you have raised the issue. A complete mental status test for refining the patient's ability, and for establishing a baseline is more appropriately a part of the neurological examination.

A complete database, including a comprehensive medical history, if one is not already available, needn't be done in one visit. Often it can be spread out over several visits, supplemented with questionnaires filled out at home.

Interviewing in the hospital or outpatient offices is little different than with younger patients, other than needing to allow extra time and offering nursing assistance in disrobing. Be alert to the possibility of the patient falling if unattended.

☐ THE HOME VISIT

Despite the general belief that house calls are a thing of the past, many physicians see patients in their homes. With older persons often lacking transportation, or being confined to bed, a house call is the only practical way to see the patient. Working in partnership with a Visiting Nurse or Nurse Practitioner is an entirely satisfactory way to provide continuity of care. Don't lightly pass up the chance to make a home visit yourself, however. Few occasions to establish rapport equal a house call. On one occasion, I visited a patient in a small town about 40 minutes from the hospital. She and her elderly sister had tea waiting, and after I took care of her medical needs, I was ushered into the dining room where her finest dishes and linen had been set and a delicious meal was waiting. Later, my visit was reported in the local weekly newspaper.

Just as important as the strengthening of rapport is the health-related information you gather while in the home. Meeting those who live with the patient, identifying safety hazards, judging the patient's capacity for activities of daily living are easily done, and often invaluable. In one case, an elderly man had been admitted to the hospital every two or three months for medication-related complications. A visit to the home revealed chaos in the medicine cabinet. Order was established, and a plan for taking medicines worked out. The patient has not been hopsitalized in the two years since the home visit. In another case, the reason for a substantial weight loss was quickly linked to the patient's inability to manage kitchen utensils because of worsening arthritis.

☐ THE TELEPHONE

The telephone is often an alternative to an office visit. You may occasionally assist the patient to obtain essential telephone service by certifying to the phone company or welfare agency the need. You should be familiar with special telephones for persons with hearing impairment and devices that automatically summon emergency help in the case of sudden disability.

☐ Difficult Relationships

Older patients frequently are considered "difficult." Often the difficulty can be traced to not knowing the circumstances that lead to behavior that is labeled as difficult.

An older man with a neurological disorder was told of the need for a lumbar puncture, to which he agreed. When a fourth year medical student appeared to do the procedure, the patient became angry and refused to cooperate, asking instead for the attending physician. Tactful questioning revealed that the patient's wife, who also had a neurological disease, had recently gone to the Mayo Clinic for treatment. His objection: "My wife gets this test at the Mayo Clinic: here I get a student!"

A man in his 60s, a retired executive, was admitted to the hospital for coronary artery disease. He was well-liked by the medical staff; his attending physician called him a "real sweetie." The nurses didn't think so, however. They found him to be demanding. And sometimes he urinated in bed. Some of the staff thought he did so deliberately.

What was happening was this: he was given a sedative at night because of trouble sleeping in the hospital environment. The first night of sedation he became confused and disoriented, and was found roaming the hospital corridors. Therefore, restraints were ordered. When the patient needed to urinate, he called to be released from the restraints. His calls were ignored, and finally he could not keep from voiding in bed. The nurse who finally came was furious, and told the others about it. Each evening thereafter he was ignored when he called for anything, and most evenings he wet the bed.

What he had learned is what every young child learns: any kind of behavior, even misbehavior, gets attention and is preferable to being ignored. If control is taken away, they find ways to get it back. Being "difficult" is one form of control.

Some patients with whom you feel uncomfortable may represent for you distressing concepts. You may see the patient as you may someday be—old and facing death.

□ Interviewing the Family

In geriatric practice, a family is often the primary source of information and planning for future care. (If no family member is available, sometimes the patient is happy to have a good friend speak with you, but *get the patient's permission* first.) In most instances, meet with both together briefly, then if at all possible talk alone with the patient. The son or daughter who accompanies the parent may be part of the problem. The patient needs an opportunity to speak confidentially. You should speak with the relative also, but let your patient know you are doing so and ask permission. The principle is that of preserving the patient's autonomy and sense of self as an independent person. Family members, with good intent, often forget that decisions should involve the person about whom the decision is made.

In one recent instance in my practice, a daughter, whose aging parents lived in another city and were having some difficulty in managing their daily activities, decided her parents would be better off living close by. She genuinely wanted to help her parents. She rented a nice apartment for them near her home, and made other arrangements for their comfort. But the move was a disaster. For her parents the move meant the loss of friendships and community organizations where they were known and had a familiar role.

Be prepared for some rough times. Relatives may be angry at you for the condition and circumstances of a parent. In some instances they may be displacing onto you their guilt and anger at having an unwanted burden, and hope to transfer that responsibility to the doctor or hospital. One woman said, "I can't accept her as my mother any more—I wish she were dead." She was angry at the doctors for keeping her mother alive. With people living well into their 80's and 90's, a son or daughter may be 60 or 70. They see in their parent themselves in the not-too-distant future. By ignoring a parent's situation, they deny their own aging.

□ Facing Death

Some older persons face the inevitability of death with more composure than do their physicians. When the physician is uneasy about death an unnecessary breakdown in communication about both practical and philosophical matters results. Among the questions that most older persons should consider are:

□ Concern for the welfare of a surviving spouse or other family member.
□ Disposal of property.
□ Wishes about heroic attempts to continue life.
□ Patients may want to sign a *Living Will* setting forth their wish to die in dignity.
□ Preferences about funeral arrangements, religious and memorial services.

Most older persons are quite prepared to face these issues, but need their physician's help. There is no better way to acknowledge these concerns than to include them as a routine part of your initial history-taking.

□ REFERENCES AND READINGS

Beresford TP, Holt RE, Hll RC, et al: Cognitive screening at the bedside: Usefulness of a structured examination. Psychosomatics 1985;26:319–324.
Burton JR, Hazzard WR: Geriatric medicine: Special considerations. *In* Barker LR, Burton JR,

Zieve PD: Principles of Ambulatory Medicine, ed 2. Baltimore, Williams & Wilkins, 1986, Chap 6.

Cadieux RJ, Kales JD, Zimmerman L: Comprehensive assessment of the elderly patient. Am Fam Physican 1985;31:105–111.

Council on Scientific Affairs, American Medical Assn: Elder abuse and neglect. JAMA 1987; 257:966–971.

Hedley R, Ebrahim DM, Sheldon M: Opportunities for anticipatory care with the elderly. J Fam Pract 1986;22:141–145.

Kane RL, Ouslander JG, Abrass IB: Evaluating the elderly, in Essentials of Clinical Geriatrics. New York, McGraw-Hill, 1984, pp 35–55.

Steel K: History taking from elderly patients. Hospital Practice 1985;30:70–71.

Steel K, Markson EW: Approach to the older patient: The diagnostic process, in Andres R, Bierman EL, Hazzard WR: Principles of Geriatric Medicine. New York, McGraw-Hill, Ch 16.

The elderly: What they really want from you (Panel discussion). Med Econ, Apr 29, 1985:44–46.

Wooliscroft JO, Calhoun JG, et al: Medical education in facilities for the elderly. JAMA 1984;252:3382–3385.

CHAPTER **24**

THE SEXUAL HISTORY
Peter J. Attarian, PhD*

Sexuality, as a component of health living, must be considered in any Health Promotion interview. Sexuality is a factor in many Problem-Centered situations, both as cause of some illnesses, and as one element in the overall treatment plan of the ill person. Sexual dysfunction as a problem in itself leads patients to seek your help. Finally, concern and fear about AIDS and other sex-related diseases, and issues such as abortion, rape, child molestation, and pornography spread to other aspects of life such as employment, school attendance, and fundamental human rights. The medical profession once all but ignored sexual matters; today, avoiding such areas is not possible without weakening the health care professional's role.

☐ Student Roles and Attitudes

The key to dealing helpfully with the sexuality of patients is being comfortable with our own sexuality. Although you may not have achieved total

*Associate Professor and Associate Head, Department of Family and Community Medicine, and Assistant Professor, Department of Psychiatry, University of Arizona College of Medicine, Tucson, Arizona

226

sexual maturity, what is important is your willingness to explore your attitudes, identify areas of strength and weakness, and find avenues of personal growth.

Beyond your level of sexual maturity are your beliefs about sexuality in general. Moral tenets and sexual practices are closely linked. Some health care providers are unable to deal objectively with homosexuality, abortion, premarital or extramarital sex, or prostitution. Prescribing artificial birth control also conflicts with some clinicians' personal principles.

Self-knowledge is the key to identifying issues that might impair your objectivity as a clinician. Most medical schools have required or elective courses in human sexuality. Community resources include workshops and discussion groups. Churches offer a variety of programs designed to promote healthy sexual growth. Finally, personal counseling is successful in correcting deep-seated difficulties that, uncorrected, have the potential for creating real difficulties in one's professional or personal life.

□ Seeking Care

□ MAKING THE APPOINTMENT

When you are in practice you will want to think about how patients arrange appointments. Will the routine of making an appointment inhibit those who are embarrassed or unwilling to tell the receptionist why an appointment is requested? If people in the waiting room can overhear everything said at the reception desk, sexual concerns are not likely to be stated. Instead, "a cold" or some other medical problem may be given as the reason for the visit. An alert staff will perceive the patient's hidden agenda. If a patient seems uncomfortable or vague about asking for an appointment, or gives as a reason "Something personal to talk to the doctor about," that should end the intake questioning.

□ PATIENT ATTITUDES

Despite the openness of sexual discussion today compared to even a decade ago, many patients still find it difficult to mention sexual concerns, even in the privacy of a clinical interview. Misinformation, rigid attitudes, guilt, and shame often hamper communication. Take nothing for granted when obtaining a sexual history. Patients often need no more than information to solve a problem, but it is up to you to assess their need correctly.

Denial may be present. The patient may not recognize the sexual basis for a medical problem, which is translated into bodily symptoms. Consider the question of sexual adjustment in working with patients whose medical problem is not clearly the result of some medical condition.

Guilt and self-imposed punishment, often out of proportion to the event, are frequently the basis of a patient seeking your help. Guilt may take many forms, including a hypochondriacal concern of having some dreaded disease such as syphilis or AIDS.

Ninety percent of patients who do seek medical care for a sexual problem will be women, frequently women who have accepted the male, "It's your problem" myth. A good question to ask yourself in *any* clinical situation is: Who is the patient? The person who makes the appointment is only one member of a dysfunctional unit, sometimes the healthier but weaker member. Empowerment of the weaker member is a key element in any type of marital/sexual counseling. Giving each partner equal time and attention can initiate major changes in a relationship.

Having both partners in a stressful sexual relationship present at some point is often helpful. Sometimes only in the safety of a third person will honest communication take place. It may be appropriate, with the patient's permission, to send a note or make a call inviting the other person to enter into the therapy.

☐ Rapport

The sexual history, sensitively done, strengthens rapport. The basics of open communication, active listening, honesty, and leadership demonstrate to the patient your competence and ability to understand needs that are difficult to express. A neutral, nonjudgmental attitude of acceptance is essential, but it is difficult to maintain if a patient's behavior conflicts with your personal values. Accepting the patient "as is" is a starting point from which to work towards sexual health. Active listening is especially important to detect the presence of a sexually related issue. Your sensitivity to the existence of a sexual "hidden agenda," or your skill in seeing beyond somatic complaints or denial may be all that is necessary to start the communication process. Detecting nonverbal clues helps, but sometimes you must intuitively sense what is on the patient's mind.

Humor aids rapport; helping the patient see a lighter side to serious problems puts problems in perspective. Humor must be appropriate; misused, the patient may misunderstand and feel put down.

☐ The Problem-Centered Interview

☐ SEXUAL DYSFUNCTION

An essential perspective in dealing with sexual difficulties is that sexuality reflects four basic dimensions:

1. Self-esteem.
2. Quality of the relationship between sexual partners.

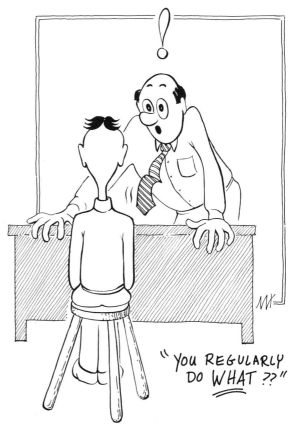

"YOU REGULARLY DO WHAT ??"

A non-judgmental attitude is essential.

3. Communication between partners.
4. Personality patterns.

Someone lacking healthy self-esteem may feel unworthy and unable to accept the love of another. When one partner in a relationship takes the other as no more than an object, sex becomes exploitation. Identifying the personality pattern of a patient gives a good clue to the kind of sexual response that person is likely to feel comfortable with, and the kinds of problems that may arise. For example, a person who is basically passive will feel comfortable with a partner who is sexually assertive, but will have difficulty if the other person is also passive. A person whose personality is generally hostile often incorporates hurtful behavior in sexual relationships. Given the range of human personality styles, the variability in sexual practice from one couple to another is enormous; knowing the basic personality style of the patient is a powerful assist in identifying sexual dysfunction. Given the assumption that sexuality is a reflection of basic interpersonal and intrapersonal processes, assessment of a patient's sexual adjustment must be looked at in a total context, not just a matter of sexual mechanics.

□ Sexual Aspects of Medical Problems

Many illnesses have sexual implications. Impotency is a common side effect of conditions such as diabetes mellitus, vascular disease, extensive prostate surgery, and some medications. Anxiety about sexual capability is a common sequelae to myocardial infarction, mastectomy, hysterectomy, or other major medical and surgical conditions. Diminished or absent libido accompanies depression. The patient recovering from a myocardial infarction, for example, may believe that any sexual arousal will overtax the heart and do further damage—a belief which in itself cripples libido. Whenever possible—before surgery or prescribing medications—the patient should be told of accompanying sexual implications. In this way the patient is not suddenly confronted with an additional stress, and often will have worked through the problem. Your ability to predict these matters strengthens your image as a knowledgeable and thoughtful clinician. Advice should be specific, however. To tell a patient recovering from a myocardial infarction that sexual activity can be resumed "Anytime you feel like it" is less helpful than "When you can climb two flights of stairs, you should be ready." Suggestions to modify usual sexual behavior are more acceptable when they come from a professional. For example, telling a man who should limit his energy expenditure that a side-by-side, or a supine position can be used is good advice during recuperation. Masturbation is also a suitable recommendation in some situations.

□ Health Promotion

Few areas offer a better opportunity for health promotion than sexuality. Adolescents, for example, are often in turmoil about sexual concerns but have no one to provide sound education and advice. The physician can be of great service to the young person in relieving doubts and guilt about issues concerning sexual activity. Also, the young person who is sexually active may know little or nothing about birth control; if so, there is an opportunity to prevent an unwanted pregnancy. Again, it will be up to the clinician to initiate discussion.

Almost any type of clinical visit offers an appropriate opportunity. A 17-year-old student coming for a routine "sports OK" may be surprised but appreciative about an inquiry like, "Sometimes sexual problems are a problem for teens. Anything you'd like to discuss?" Even though the answer is a brief, "No problem," you have established yourself as an interested and thoughtful person. Weeks or months later the patient may return to discuss his or her sexual questions.

Some patients may not anticipate questions about sexuality as a part of obtaining a Health Promotion database. No one approach is suitable for all patients. Usually all that is needed is a simple statement about the fact that sexual matters are a part of health, followed by an open-ended question, such as:

"How do you feel about your sexual life?"

"Is sex a problem for you?"

"Are you sexually active?"

There is a hierachy of questioning levels. "Normal" sexuality may be easily discussed on the first visit, but queries about possibly deviant or harmful activities such as incest or other sexual activity require considerable trust before such issues can safely be brought out into the open. For sensitive matters the patient is not yet ready to discuss, it is helpful to make a comment indicating that you are open to discussion sometimes in the future, such as

"I think it is an important matter—we should discuss it sometime."

The use of questionnaires or personal diaries assists communication about problems a patient may be unable to discuss openly (*see Chapter 29: Checklists, Questionnaires, and Forms*). Similarly, sensitivity to the patient's acceptance of professional associates, such as the office nurse, who assists in data gathering is required. Patients who barely have the courage to tell you of their sexual problem may be completely unable to tell someone else. And, of course, all history-taking must be done in a secure place, out of hearing range of others.

Sometimes you may sense that a particular patient would be offended by any inquiry about sexual matters, and decide to omit the issue, at least for the time being. Usually, however, you will be surprised by how easy, and even welcome, such questioning is.

□ Prevention

For a couple about to start a family, parenting classes are invaluable in providing practical guidance about the many challenges of raising children, including developing a healthy attitude about their sexuality. If parents are shy or uncomfortable with their sexuality, if rigid and unenlightened dogma or taboos permeate the home, or if sex isn't talked about, a child raised in this environment may later acquire misinformation and unwholesome attitudes. The end result is too often a perpetuation of an unsatisfactory sexual orientation. It is the parent's role to foster healthy sexuality in their children, but parents may first need help with their own attitudes and information.

The *premarital examination* and its special importance in preparing persons about to be married for the challenges of living together is discussed in *Chapter 12: The Health Promotion Interview.*

□ Interviewing Techniques

□ VERBAL COMMUNICATION

What language is appropriate in discussing sexual matters? Should vernacular ever be used, for example? My approach is to use straightforward anatomical terms and avoid jargon or highly technical medical terms. You must, of course, constantly monitor your patient's understanding. If an unfamiliar term is used, and the patient seems confused, explain what you mean before continuing.

Different kinds of questioning skills provide different kinds of information. Direct questions about sexual practices may not be answered if put in a 'Yes or no" format. "Do you masturbate?" may cause a patient to be defensive; asking, "How often do you masturbate?" carries no value judgment with it. The patient is free to say "I don't," but also free to give a positive answer from which further discussion is possible. Open-ended questions are valuable, such as

"Tell me about a sexual experience that was troubling for you."

Role playing is a useful skill in some situations. For example, a patient may say that getting the partner to participate in therapy is an impossibility. In such a situation, ask the patient to consider you as the absent partner. Establish a dialogue that explores the sexual problem and enlists the partner's cooperation.

Finally, I try not to lose sight of the fact that patients are *people* and their difficulties are *problems*, not *cases*. It does matter how you think about patients. If, for example, you are seeing someone who is troubled about homosexual activity, to label that person as a homosexual, rather than as a person with a homosexual concern, causes a loss of human individuality and creates a barrier in your ability to be helpful.

□ Nonverbal Communication

Be alert to nonverbal clues of anxiety: behaviors such as sudden overactivity, rapid talking, or the sudden shift to abstract or intellectualized terms.

Patients with hysterical personalities are particularly liable to sexual dysfunctions. Somewhat paradoxically, they dress and behave in a seductive way, suggesting just the opposite of their true sexual adjustment. On the other hand, if someone is meticulous in all aspects of dress and behavior, speaks in a precise, controlled way, and rarely shows emotional spontaneity, you may suspect a similar pattern in sexual relationships.

□ The Interview as Therapy and Patient Education

Therapy and information are intertwined. Sometimes simply providing information is all that is necessary to relieve a patient of guilt or anxiety. Being assured that impulses or sexual practices the patient considers "evil" or "abnormal" are, in fact, neither, is often the first step in sexual growth. Near the end of every interview, or whenever I feel the patient has developed trust and a little courage, I ask, "Are there things you'd like to ask me?" This is an the invitation for the patients to reveal just what has been bothering them.

A sensitive interview in which the facts of the situation are clearly stated and received in a nonjudgmental manner puts the patients's concern in perspective and serves as guilt-relieving confession. This doesn't mean approval of whatever the patient has done. Some sexual behavior is clearly harmful to the patient and others and cannot be dismissed simply by talking about it. But sharing the problem with a thoughtful person lessens feelings of isolation, decreases self-condemnation, and sets in motion remedial activities.

□ Difficult Relationships and Special Situations

Difficult situations in sexual counseling often arise, as they do elsewhere, when you have not achieved the necessary degree of objectivity. Common responses are either moving away, or moving towards the patient. Avoiding the issues is the easiest "out," even in the presence of unmistakable signals that the patient is asking for help. Intellectualization—giving facts or providing reading material, but not dealing with the patient's feelings—is another way of sidestepping helpful discussion.

Inappropriately moving towards the patient is also not helpful. Lecturing or moralizing, or creating a punishing or guilt-laden interaction, does not alter patients' behavior, but does impair rapport. Satisfying your personal curiosity in the guise of an excessively detailed history is inconsistent with the professional relationship. Some physicians have carried self-deception to an extreme by developing a personal sexual relationship with a patient, rationalizing that such behavior is "therapeutic" for the patient.

The mistaken identity issues discussed in *Chapter 20: Difficult Relationships* may influence how you perceive your patient, and the kind of advice you offer. Too closely identifying with a patient, for example, may result in recommending solutions that work for you but that are not necessarily appropriate for the patient.

Patients may lose their objectivity about you and, consciously or unconsciously, try to turn a professional relationship into a personal one. Questions about your marital status or overtly seductive behaviors often signal a hidden agenda. Should a patient who uses the medical setting to express sexual difficulties happen to have a physician who also has unresolved sexual problems, the potential for mutually harmful interaction is great.

□ REFERENCES AND READINGS

Blume J: The Judy Blume Diary; The Place to Put Your Feelings. New York, Dell, 1981.
Comfort A: The Joy of Sex. New York, Pocket Books, 1985.
Ende J, Rockwell S, Glasgow M: The sexual history in general medicine practice. Arch Intern Med 1984;144:558–561.
Frolkis JP: "AIDS" anxiety. Postgrad Med 1986;79:265–276.
Kaplan HS: New Sex Therapy, Active Treatment of Sexual Dysfunctions. New York, Times Books, 1974.
Kentsmith, DK, Eaton MT: Treating Sexual Problems in Medical Practice. New York, Arco Publishing, 1979.
Lief HI (ed): Sexual Problems in Medical Practice. Chicago, American Medical Association, 1981.
Nadelson CC, Marcotte DB: Treatment Interventions in Human Sexuality. New York, Plenum Press, 1983.
Pariser SF, Levine SG, Gardner ML (eds): Clinical Sexuality. New York, Marcel Dekker, 1983.
Payton CE: Sexual counseling. In Taylor RE (ed): Family Medicine: Principles and Practice, ed 2. New York, Springer-Verlag, 1983, pp 219–236.
Woods NF: Human Sexuality in Health and Illness. St. Louis, C.V. Mosby, 1984, Chap 5.

CHAPTER 25

VIP'S, FAMILY, AND FRIENDS

The first chapter in this unit emphasized that the quality of the doctor-patient relationship is a function of the individual qualities of each person. Exceptional relationships are sometimes the most revealing about our patients, and ourselves. Taking care of VIP's (Very Important People), while infrequent in most practices, offers special challenges to the professional relationship. Similarly, caring for family members, close friends, or physicians is rarely a routine experience.

☐ The VIP

Persons with special status, power, wealth, or influence get sick like everyone else. Many VIP's are mature persons who create no special problems when they need medical attention. But others have purchased their success at a substantial personal cost. These persons seem driven to excel. And once they have succeeded, they find themselves driven still harder to retain what they have, or to climb higher. Many of these people, despite their accomplishments, suffer from a basic insecurity or a fear of failure that cannot be quieted by their extraordinary efforts.

When such persons enter the sick role, a number of stresses are likely to arise. Illness serious enough to interrupt their daily routine means loss of control and an enforced awareness of their personal vulnerability. VIPs do not easily relinquish control of their life pattern to their caretakers, however necessary such accommodations are to adequate care. Nor do they deal comfortably with questions about aspects of their personal lives they wish to conceal. Excessive use of alcohol, use of illicit drugs, or risky sexual practices, all having medical relevance, may be consciously evaded or unconsciously denied. A VIP who has lived in an environment of interpersonal manipulations in exchange for favors may expect caretakers to do the same, resulting in mistrust of genuine caring and an unselfish wish to help. In other words, the style and personality patterns of some VIP's make caring for them a difficult, thankless task.

☐ Collusion of the Physician

When you add the human weaknesses of caretakers to the personality characteristics of some VIP's, the resulting loss of objectivity sets the stage for inadequate care. There are special factors that may distort a physician's professional judgment.

Caring for a notable person implies special personal or professional qualities that further one's career. To avoid threatening the relationship, the physician may make unwise exceptions and compromises. A successful medical outcome may lead the VIP to bestow special favors on the physician. While these may be of a material nature, they may also be recommendations to important positions in the community, financial advice, or opening the doors of exclusive clubs or organizations.

The other side of the coin is the consequences of failure. Should care not go entirely to the satisfaction of the VIP, the physician may be subjected to unusual pressures, either directly in terms of being dismissed or indirectly through pressure from hospital administrators or senior physicians. Given the prospect of gain if things go well, and loss if things go not well, two reactions are likely. One common reaction is *overtreatment* in terms of excessive tests and consultations to ensure that "nothing is missed," and over-aggressive therapies to cover all possibilities. Sometimes, too, there is a temptation to provide care beyond the physician's usual area of expertise when ordinarily a referral would have been made.

The other inappropriate response is *undertreatment*. This may take the form of not asking about potentially embarrassing aspects of the patient's medical history during the interview, failing to perform unpleasant or uncomfortable examinations, such as a rectal examination or a sigmoidoscopy, ordering minimal or excessively conservative treatment, or avoiding the patient altogether.

Mr. J., a millionaire, contributed a small fortune to the local medical school. In appreciation, the school named a new hospital wing after him. Several years later he needed elective surgery, and was admitted to the hospital wing bearing his name.

No medical student was assigned to the case of this "private patient." The junior resident assumed that, naturally, the chief resident would look after such a prestigious person. The chief resident assumed that the attending physician would assume the responsibility. The attending physician had other things on his mind. Mr. J. suffered from not-so-benign neglect for several days until the head nurse pointed out to all concerned what was happening.

□ Caring for Family and Friends

Family members and friends, when accepted as patients, pose some of the same obstacles as caring for VIP's. The wish for hero status may make it difficult to admit that you really are not the physician to care for some condition outside your usual area of competence. A natural wish to maintain a positive relationship may conflict with the demands of good care. This often includes overlooking shortcomings that, if disclosed, would be a threat to the other's self-esteem. You may want to exempt your friend or family member from unpleasantness or discomfort. To confront a patient with the fact of alcoholism is one thing; to confront a family member or close friend who is an alcoholic is another. And, as with caring for the VIP, if things do not go well, personal reproach and guilt may result. Although there are times when you feel comfortable about caring for family or friends, in most instances you best serve those who are emotionally close to you by arranging for appropriate care—by someone else.

□ Caring for Colleagues

Physicians, as a group, receive notoriously inadequate medical treatment. Caring for colleagues is another variation on the VIP theme. Being selected to provide care by a member of one's profession implies a high regard for your medical competence. But the need to accommodate to the physician/patient and maintain cordial relations leads to departure from standards of routine care, usually undertreatment.

A physician recently consulted a leading urologist because of chronic prostatitis. The urologist took a detailed history, but failed to perform the most fundamental step in physical examination of the prostate, the rectal examination.

Undertreatment may result from another cause: lack of payment. Traditionally, physicians extend to colleagues professional courtesy in the form of free care. The physician/patient, anticipating this professional courtesy, ends up informally asking medical advice in the hospital coffee shop or in the corridor to avoid causing the other economic loss. Also, the person wishing help feels an obligation to minimize the demands on the friend and avoids becoming yet another patient on a busy schedule.

Perhaps the single greatest obstacle to receiving adequate care is denial.

An internist who specialized in studying the psychological behavior of patients with coronary artery disease was addressing a group of cardiologist when he himself suffered a major myocardial infarction. Cardiopulmonary resuscitation was successfully administered by one of the cardiologists. Later, the physician/patient admitted that he had been experiencing angina pectoris for several years, but had ignored the symptom.

For almost a week a highly competent gastroenterologist noted with mild curiosity that his stools were black—almost certainly a sign of gastrointestinal bleeding. He felt well, however, and did nothing to investigate the condition. Then he experienced brief episodes of faintness and was alarmingly pale. He finally consulted an associate (while the two were riding up in a hospital elevator). The presence of active gastrointestinal bleeding from a tear in the esophagus, a condition he had often diagnosed in others, was soon established.

The origins of denial among physicians are the result of many factors, including knowing too much about the possibility of serious disease, not wishing to appear foolish for letting the self-neglect go on, and the sense of invincibility that comes with successfully caring for patients. Whatever the cause, the old dictum about "He who cares for himself has a fool for a doctor," applies.

Two specific steps that minimize the dangers associated for the "special" treatment accorded physicians are: obtain adequate health insurance throughout your career (starting as a student), and see a physician who doesn't know you personally. When you are rich and/or famous, and in need of expert medical care, your best bet may be to go to a distant city where you are not known, and do not divulge that you are a physician. Sign in as "Mr." or "Mrs." rather than as "Dr." Most of all, don't enter the health care system expecting extraordinary attention—you might get it.

□ Confidentiality

An inherent risk to any prominent person who needs medical attention is gossip. However committed health care providers are to the principles of confidentiality, irresponsible and sometimes damaging gossip does take place. This subject is discussed in the next chapter.

□ Conclusion

This chapter is filled with warnings about caring for VIP's and others with whom an exceptional relationship is present. This doesn't mean that you should avoid caring for such persons altogether, only that you look deeply into yourself and understand your human weaknesses as well as your strengths. An honest relationship with a close friend or prominent person may result in great benefit. Indeed, think of the VIP as a Very Important *Patient* with human needs the same as anyone else, but whose very accomplishments have resulted in a special kind of isolation that makes a helping relationship difficult to maintain.

□ REFERENCES AND READINGS

Baron RJ: An introduction to medical phenomenology. I can't hear you while I am talking. Ann Intern Med 1985;103:606–611.

Doctors as patients: Not always too patient. Med World News 1986; July 28:42–57.

Pinner M, Miller BF: When Doctors are Patients. New York, WW Norton, 1952.

Scott CD, Hawk J: Heal Thyself: The Health Care of Professionals. New York, Brunner/Mazel, 1986.

The VIP. Audio-Digest Family Practice, Vol 26, no. 33, Sept 4, 1978.

What you can learn from doctors who are patients (panel discussion). Modern Medicine 1985; Sept:60–71.

UNIT VII

COMMUNICATION WITHIN THE PROFESSION

CHAPTER 26

CONFIDENTIALITY

> ... And whatsoever I shall see or hear in the course of my profession, as well as outside my profession in my intercourse with men, if it be what should not be published abroad, I will never divulge, holding such things to be holy secrets.
>
> *Hippocrates*

☐ Gossip

As you interview patients, you are often privileged to share in patients' personal thoughts, feelings, and behaviors. Patients who share sensitive information with you expect you to use it discreetly, repeating it only in the interest of their health goals. When personal information is shared with others who have no right to it, the danger of harm exists.

I was hosting a small dinner, and among those invited was Arthur T, who had been in the headlines recently because of a political controversy.

A few days before the party I was discussing the controversy with an acquaintance. At one point he said, "Too bad about Arthur T, I understand he has cancer and doesn't have too long to live." I knew nothing about this illness; in fact, when he accepted the dinner invitation Arthur sounded as vigorous as ever. But when I heard the same story a second time from another person, I expected Arthur to arrive in an ambulance, if he arrived at all. In fact, he looked the picture of health, and had second helpings of everything. If he had cancer, he was tolerating it with exceptional strength and good spirits.

When I heard the rumor a third time I decided to track down its source. What happened was that Arthur had recently had a small mole excised. The pathological report was equivocal, as is sometimes the case, concluding that a

243

malignant melanoma could not be definitely ruled out. The specimen was then referred to several pathologists who were expert in diagnosing melanoma; all agreed that the lesion was benign. In the meantime, however, someone in the hospital who saw the initial report mentioned the fact of a possible melanoma to his wife, who relayed the story to others, omitting the word "possible."

Fortunately, the rumor did no harm. Arthur had a good laugh when I told him about it. However, at the time he was negotiating an important career change and promotion, which did go through successfully. I couldn't help wondering, however, had the rumor spread and adversely affected his career, whether the hospital could have been successfully sued. In any event, the rumor could have been harmful to a patient who expected the medical profession to be for him, not against him.

☐ VIP's

Well-known persons are especially vulnerable to gossip, especially when the news is negative or suggests moral misconduct. Nobody seems to care if the mayor is admitted for an appendectomy, but should the same person have a venereal disease, an alcohol problem, or incurable cancer, the word travels quickly. Physicians and nurses are not exempt from gossip when receiving care in the hospital or clinic where they work and are well known. Perhaps deep in the reaches of human nature is a dark trait that enjoys seeing well-known persons experience adversity. Or maybe the reason why VIP's privacy is violated is the indirect ego-boost associated with caring for a person of status. Whatever the reason, spreading bad news about well-known persons happens often, even when there is no conscious intent to harm the person involved.

☐ The Need to Share

There are times when you will need to discuss difficult problems with a trusted friend or spouse. A good rule is not to identify the patient you are discussing by name. No matter how carefully the information is given and received, leaks occur. When more than one person knows a secret, it no longer is a secret. Also, the person receiving the information may be placed in an uncomfortable situation when meeting the person about whom confidential information is known. Pretending not to know is often revealing to a perceptive person.

☐ Charts and Other Hazards

Medical records are a frequent source of breaches of confidentiality. The paper-based unit record used in almost all health care facilities passes through many hands and before many eyes. Before writing anything sensitive in a chart, consider who might have access to your comments.

You will also want to think about the possibility of the patient, or a relative of the patient, overhearing what you are saying. The hospital cafeteria, the nurses' station, and outpatient facilities lend themselves to careless communication.

CHAPTER 27

27

RECORDS AND WRITTEN COMMUNICATIONS

Problem-Oriented Medical
  Record (POMR)
Graphic Representations
Multiple Problems
Forms
Clarity
Verbiage
Communicating with Other
  Physicians
Legal Implications

The information you acquire during the interview is of little value until it is recorded. The medical record is the final destination of the medical history. Just as record keeping is essential in the operation of all types of businesses, from banks to airlines, so is it an integral part of the health care process. Once recorded, the patient's clinical history is available to all members of the health care team, is immune to the loss and distortion of memory, and can be constantly reviewed, evaluated, and updated. The record is an indispensable tool that guides your thoughts and actions.

The record supports a wide variety of clinical tasks:

☐ Problem-centered care.
☐ Health promotion.
☐ Coordinating activities of the health care team.
☐ Alerting the health care team to high-risk situations.
☐ Evaluation (audit) of care.
☐ Detection of trends in disease in the community.
☐ Cost containment.
☐ Research and teaching.

☐ Problem-Oriented Medical Record (POMR)

The POMR is a system of medical record keeping introduced by Dr. Lawrence Weed (Hurst, 1972). Until the development of the POMR, the typical record was a disorganized volume of information that lacked page numbers, a table of contents, and an index. The POMR assigns consecutive numbers to each of a patient's medical conditions, and creates a numbered *Problem List* that acts as a table of contents. New information entered into the chart is

246

labeled by problem name and corresponding number. Each clinical note is structured by a *SOAP* format, the initials referring to *S*ubjective and *O*bjective data, *A*ssessment, and *P*lans. Plans are categorized according to purpose: diagnosis (further testing), therapy, and patient education.

Another innovation of the POMR is grouping information according to the problem. In the past, each health care provider, such as physician, nurse, or social worker, entered comments in a separate section of the record, contributing to fragmentation of information.

Any form of record keeping demands a certain amount of organized thinking before an entry is made. The POMR format makes you think in an orderly, logical fashion about what is going on with the patient and what you plan to do. It uncovers gaps in your knowledge, and directs you to areas that need more information.

The POMR, despite the logic of its format, has not been widely implemented. Old patterns of charting are difficult to break. The POMR requires substantial relearning, and takes added effort to maintain. Nor does the POMR overcome the difficulties created by illegible writing, misplaced charts, or unauthorized access to confidential information. (The role of the computer in solving these shortcomings is discussed in the next Unit.) Given the pressures of practice, and the traditional view of charting as a necessary evil rather than a valuable clinical tool, it is not surprising that the POMR has received a mixed reception. Whether or not your school or clinical sites use the POMR, become familiar with the POMR *concept* of organizing data. The POMR is more than a system of record keeping; it is a rational, disciplined way of thinking about patient care.

□ Graphic Representations

The medical record is primarily a text document, but at times graphs, tables, and flow charts illustrate relationships that are not evident from the text alone. Charting variables like vital signs, laboratory test results, and medications is the only easy way to see at a glance the overall situation of patients with conditions such as diabetes mellitus, hypertension, and other chronic diseases. Charting a patient's health history on a time line indicating important life events often makes clear psychosocial relationships. A patient may report, at various times during an interview, the following:

". . .divorced when I was 30."
". . .mother died in 1970."
". . .had my first bout with ulcers about 16 years ago."

By plotting these events on a single dated line the clustering of events becomes evident. It takes a bit of calculating to determine the year he was divorced and what year he first had ulcers, but if the data from the patient are accurate, useful correlations emerge. In addition to events in a patient's personal life, you may notice correlations with economic recessions, wars, the fortunes of the local baseball team, or maybe even sunspots.

☐ Multiple Problems

Unit II: Problem-Solving focused on the diagnostic process applied to a single clinical problem. The realities of daily medical care, however, involve caring for people with multiple problems. Patients may have several independent diseases like osteoarthritis and asthma, or related problems like hypertension and heart failure. Commonly, medications used for one condition create problems for another condition: for example, diuretics that control hypertension may cause digitalis used in treating heart failure to become toxic. Further, a physician preoccupied with caring for multiple active problems may overlook the patient's less urgent but no less important health promotion needs. To cite just one instance: an effective pneumococcal vaccine has been administered to only a fraction of persons at high risk because of chronic lung disease, alcoholism, immune deficiencies, and other conditions that predispose to pneumococcal pneumonia.

The structure of traditional records obscures the existence of multiple problems and overlapping therapies. The Problem List of the POMR format is one answer; it shows at a glance all the patient's active problems. When the POMR is combined with a computer that actively highlights omissions and risk situations, the record then supports the highest quality comprehensive health care.

☐ Forms

Some records start off as blank sheets, to be structured by the clinician. More often, the record consists of preprinted database forms, plus blank sheets for progress notes. Forms help the information management process by listing the information requirements of a database, which ensures completeness of data collection.

Forms have one major disadvantage: they encourage passive data collection. The temptation is great to turn the interview into a passive "filling in the blanks" session. The objections to using forms to guide your interview *while you are a student* are substantial:

☐ You will never become a skilled interviewer able to adapt to the uniqueness of each patient.

☐ Forms vary in their quality. Some hospitals and outpatient facilities use forms which are thoughtfully prepared by a committee of local physicians. Other facilities, however, use commercially prepared forms, some of which appear to be decades old. To meet the needs of a broad base of customers, they either are so complete they are unwieldy, or so general they are of little value.

□ When you enter practice, where using forms may be appropriate, you will lack the interviewing experience needed to design a form specifically suited to your needs and clinical style.

□ Clarity

Physicians' chart write-ups are rarely literary gems. Often they are disasters of redundancy (. . . on auscultation a murmur is heard), cliches (well-developed, well-nourished white male in no acute distress), verbiage (The patient comes to the clinic today with a complaint of . . .) or repetition (. . . diarrhea for 2 weeks. The initial episode started 2 weeks ago . . .). In addition to these errors are grammatical flaws that carry medical jargon and cliches to ridiculous extremes:

"The patient lost 1000 cc of blood on the table."

"The surgeon under general anesthesia removed the gallbladder."

"The patient was discharged, to be followed by a small bowel series."

"She had mild depression from viewing her chart."

"The patient was seen by this examiner who was having contractions."

"The wound was placed at bed rest."

"The patient gets nauseated after intercourse which lasts six or seven hours."

Lack of planning or carelessness when writing or dictating results in wasted time (yours and whoever reads your notes) and wasted money paid to medical transcriptionists who must type out the nonsense. Most important, however, is that sloppy communication creates patient care problems. No one can accurately remember all the details of a patient's health history from one visit to the next; the record is indispensable. Also, other members of the health care team cannot learn about the patient if the record is disorganized, sketchy, or illegible.

□ Verbiage

At least half the words of the average chart entry could be eliminated with no loss of meaning. The following chart entry, taken from an actual outpatient record, demonstrates common flaws that obscure medical communication. The notes have then been rewritten in a tight, telegraphic style. The original entry has about 400 words; the rewrite about 150 words. Knowing what to include and what to omit is partly a function of experience, but you can be reasonably brief if a few moments are spent organizing your thoughts before writing.

☐ PROGRESS NOTES (ORIGINAL)

Date & Time:
Patient Name and Number:

cc: Vomiting and diarrhea past 2 wks
Wt: 81 kgs.   B/P: 112/64 LAS   Temp: 37
The patient presents with a chief complaint of vomiting and diarrhea for the past two weeks. The initial episode started two weeks ago when the patient had onset of diarrhea and fever which lasted for five days. This was accompanied by a fever. The patient characterized the diarrhea as watery with no formed element, no gas, no blood. This subsided for approximately three or four days, and then recurred again with onset of vomiting later followed by diarrhea similar to the previous episode. This persisted for another four or five days and subsided. The patient again noted onset of symptoms yesterday but these seemed to be clearing. Patient denies any other associated symptoms. Diet during these episodes consisted mainly of clear liquids. The patient denies travel to Mexico or other areas recently. The patient states that between these episodes, his stools are normal in color and consistency. He denies any light-colored stools, abdominal pain, right upper quadrant tenderness, or change in diet recently. The only medication he was taking during this illness was PeptoBismol and no other medication. The patient has no serious chronic diseases, has been in relatively good health all his life. Patient drinks occasionally and also smokes one and a half packs of cigarettes per day. The patient is a boiler-maker by trade.

Physical exam revealed a well developed, well nourished, white male in no apparent distress. Vital signs: blood pressure is 112/64, pulse 80, temperature 37 degrees. Head, eyes, ears, nose and throat are unremarkable. The neck is without adenopathy. Thyroid is normal. Lungs: clear to A & P. Heart: normal. No murmurs detected. Abdomen is non-tender, no masses. Liver span approximately 8 cm in the midclavicular line. No spleen was palpated. There was no adenopathy in the groin area.

A: Viral gastroenteritis. The lack of systemic toxicity, bloody stools, and other symptoms speak against a bacterial etiology. Recurrent nature of this problem is probably due to incompletely healed intestinal mucosa being challenged too quickly with solid food.

P: Obtain stools for O & P and culture and sensitivity. CBC and differential with liver battery also ordered. Patient instructed to drink only clear liquids if this problem recurs and to return to a normal diet slowly following diarrhea.

Return to clinic if symptoms worsen or new problems develop.

□ REWRITE

Subjective

Present Illness. Vomiting, watery diarrhea and fever: two 5-day episodes in past two weeks—well in between with normal stool. Rx: Pepto Bismol without improvement. No abdominal or RUQ pain, light-colored or bloody stool, "gas." During diarrhea episodes, was on clear liquids. Otherwise on normal diet.

Relevant Past History: Good health, no prior GI illness.

Relevant Family History: No family or friends have similar illness.

Relevant Personal/Social History: Work: Boilermaker. Married, no children. No recent travel, change in diet. Alcohol-occasional.

Objective

B/P 112/64, P 80, T 37, Wt 81 kg
Healthy appearing, stocky built, ambulant man.
HEENT: Neg. No icterus.
Neck: No adenopathy, thyroid normal.
Heart: Normal.
Lungs: Clear to A & P.
Abd: Non-tender, no masses, liver span 8 cm/MCL, Spleen, not palp. Bowel sounds normal.

Assessment

Consistent with viral gastroenteritis, recurrent diarrhea due to incompletely healed intestinal mucosa challenged too quickly with solids. Lack of systemic toxicity, bloody stool against bacterial etiology.

Plans

DX: CBC, diff, liver profile, O & P, stool culture.
TX: Clear fluids grad. return to normal diet
Ed: Call or return if SX recur.

The many abbreviations can be a problem if not standardized. For example, "ms" can refer to "morphine sulfate," "medical student," "mitral stenosis," "multiple sclerosis," "mental status," "musculoskeletal,". . .

□ Communicating with Other Physicians

Health care teams are either formal or informal. Formal health care teams, of which you will be a part during your hospital clerkships, are composed of health care providers who interact daily within the hospital. The informal health care team is made up of the referring physician, who may not practice in the hospital to which the patient has been admitted, members of the referring physician's office staff, and community health workers such as visiting nurses and social workers. These are the people who will resume care when the patient is discharged from the hospital, yet frequently they are not informed of their patient's progress and plans for discharge. Sending regular progress notes and a discharge summary to the patient's community health care provider is both a courtesy and an obligation. University medical centers seem to have particular difficulty in keeping in touch with referring community physicians. In one study (Cummings et al, 1980) university consultants provided timely reports to the referring physician only 59 percent of the time.

Similarly, when requesting a consultation or referring a patient for hospital admission, be sure the consultant or hospital staff has a summary of the patient's condition and the questions for which a consultation or hospitalization is requested. A referral should not be a guessing game, nor should the consultant have to obtain already well-documented information. Yet the gaps in communication between physicians in different settings, and sometimes even within the same health care facility are enormous, costly, and sometimes dangerous.

An elderly woman was hospitalized by way of the emergency room following a fall that resulted in a fractured hip. Despite repeated requests of the patient and her family that her regular physician be notified of her hospitalization, this was not done, nor were her records requested. More than a week went by before her doctor learned of the admission, and only because of a call from the family. In the meantime, the patient has become seriously depressed, had developed a recurrence of a chronic condition that had been easily managed in the past, and was about to be placed on an antibiotic to which she was allergic.

□ Legal Implications

No practitioner can expect never to make a serious error, but does have the obligation to minimize the chances of mistakes occurring. A well-structured record system which guides how information is obtained and used is good insurance against charges of malpractice. It is also a valuable asset if a case comes to court. Kenneth E. Brooton, Jr. (1982), an attorney specializing in medical malpractice, advises:

Physicians who recognize that everything in the record serves a purpose have a better sense of the importance of the record in better patient care and, when necessary, in their defense. They consider record keeping an integral part of rendering care. They do not make errors that come back to haunt them on the witness stand.

□ Conclusion

Modern medical practice cannot be separated from the efficient management of information. Well-organized records and clear written communications are essential to optimal, comprehensive care. As the health care system becomes more specialized and complex, adequate communications will become an increasingly critical need.

The relationship of records to problems of confidentiality is discussed in *Chapter 26: Confidentiality.* The application of computer capabilities to medical records and communication of clinical information is discussed in *Chapter 30: Computers and Interviewing.*

□ REFERENCES AND READINGS

Brooten KE Jr: What a malpractice attorney looks for in medical records. Physician's Management 1982; November:36–40.

Cummins RO, Smith RW, Inui TS: Communication failure in primary care: Failure of consultants to provide follow-up information. JAMA 1980;243:1650–1652.

Harris ED, Lieberman, JA III: The art of consultation and referral. Medical Times 1986;114:97–100.

Hurst JW, Walker HK: The Problem Oriented System. New York, Medcom, 1972.

Levinson D: Information management in clinical practice. J Fam Pract 1978;7:799–805.

Rakel RE: Problem-oriented medical records. *In* Rakel RE (ed): Textbook of Family Practice, ed 3. Philadelphia, WB Saunders Co, 1984, pp 1363–1399.

Rakel RE: Use of consultants. *In* Rakel RE (ed): Textbook of Family Practice, ed 3. Philadelphia, WB Saunders Co, 1984, pp 190–197.

28

THE BRIEF PRESENTATION

Presenting a concise summary of patient information to others—classmates, attending physicians, consultants—is an essential clinical skill. These spoken presentations take place in a classroom, a conference hall, a busy clinic, a hospital staff room, or at the bedside. A careful and concise presentation that leaves few unanswered questions documents your clinical abilities to a far greater degree than does the written record. A few extra minutes organizing your presentation is time well invested. A rambling, poorly organized presentation is irritating, wastes time, and may obscure your overall competence in the eyes of others.

The purpose of a presentation is to communicate to the attending physician and other members of the health care team the nature of the patient's clinical problem. Sharing your knowledge about a patient enables all the team members to participate in clinical problem-solving and therapy.

☐ Content of a Brief Presentation

☐ INTRODUCTION AND PATIENT IDENTIFICATION

Identify the Patient (Name, Age, Sex, Race, Marital Status, Occupation) and mention any special circumstances about the present encounter. Comment on the patient's reliability as an index of the accuracy of the information you will give.

Subjective

1. The general nature of the problem: a *broad overall orienting statement* mentioning the major symptoms and events, usually in a chronological order.

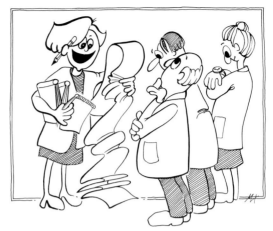

A poorly organized presentation may obscure
your overall competence.

2. If a single complaint, the *Sacred Seven* (location, quality, time patterns, severity, setting/onset, modifying factors, associated symptoms).

3. *Relevant* Past Health History: *Relevant* Family Health History and *Relevant* Personal and Social History.

4. Patient concerns.

Objective

1. A brief general *description* of the patient (avoid cliches).
2. Vital signs.
3. Relevant physical findings both positive and negative (see example).
4. Any laboratory work done so far.

Assessment

A brief interpretation of the data in terms of organ or system involved, type of pathology, and risk factors.

Plans

Plans consist of three parts:

1. *Diagnostic* plans—further diagnostic testing.
2. *Treatment* plans—may be specific, or only symptomatic, pending outcome of diagnostic tests.
3. *Patient Education*—what the patient has been told about the illness,

and what to expect or look for; what to do in case of complications; when to return; plans for future care.

□ A Brief Presentation

□ PATIENT IDENTIFICATION

Mrs. Jones is a 29-year-old, white housewife and mother of three who lives in the university area.

Each item of information helps the listener think about the patient and the kinds of diseases that are common for that age-sex-race-occupation group.

□ SUBJECTIVE DATA

Present Illness

She came to the clinic because of the rather sudden onset of sharp left anterior chest pain—just below her breast—while doing her usual housework yesterday, about 18 hours ago. The pain was severe enough to cause her to hold her side, and has been getting worse all night. Nothing helps it, and deep breathing may cause it to worsen.

The first six of the *Sacred Seven* helps "zero in on" possible systems. For a person in this age group these symptoms suggest respiratory disease. However, cardiac disease is also a possibility.

In addition to the pain, she has developed fever, an occasional cough, and a little sputum, but hasn't coughed up blood and isn't wheezing or short of breath. Last night her temperature was 103°.

Tells all you can think of to help judge the possible involvement of respiratory system. These "associated symptoms" are the Respiratory System Review. The fever suggests the *pathological process* is inflammation.

She isn't aware of any cardiac symptoms—no palpitations, irregular heart beat, orthopnea, angina-like pain, or leg edema.

The *pertinent negatives* begin the process of differential diagnosis by "ruling out" diagnostic possibilities which you considered at the onset of the clinical encounter. You are saying, in effect "Although the initial complaint might be due to a heart condition, there aren't any supportive cardiac symptoms." Lack of other cardiac symptoms doesn't eliminate the possibility—just makes it less likely.

Except for being worried that she might have a heart condition, she has no other symptoms.

A brief summary statement that tells the attending physician you've determined the limits of the Present Illness.

Past Medical History

As a child she had pneumonia twice, but no respiratory disease since the age of 12. Otherwise she has been generally healthy and was feeling well until this illness started. She has no history of rheumatic fever.

> The one past condition that might be relevant, pneumonia, is mentioned. Other illnesses (such as measles, mumps, a broken arm, or appendicitis) are not relevant and not mentioned, but are available in the comprehensive database. A common cardiac condition, rheumatic fever, which could have occurred earlier in life is specifically mentioned as a pertinent negative which further excludes the heart as the location of the disease.

Her only current medication is birth control pills; she has been on them five years without trouble and has no present leg pain or swelling.

> This indicates you've thought about the possibility of a pulmonary embolus (blood clot from legs to lungs, sometimes related to taking oral contraceptives) causing the patient's chest pain. If this possibility didn't occur to you, the attending physician might ask if you have these data.

Her last menstrual period, three weeks ago, was normal.

> Tends to rule out an early pregnancy, which would influence a decision about use of x-ray films or drugs.

She has a drug allergy to penicillin—she gets hives. She has had other antibiotics occasionally and usually develops diarrhea after a few days.

> To keep you and the patient out of trouble when prescribing treatment.

Hereditary/Contagious History, Family History

Her husband and three young children are well. Except for her father, who died of a heart attack at age 70, there is no family history of cardiac or respiratory disease. A woman she plays bridge with, however, is sick with something like the patient's illness, although she doesn't know the details.

> Indicates nothing significant in terms of hereditary illness. The bridge partner's disease might be a useful clue about a contagious disease. (Mrs. Jones' sister has multiple sclerosis; this doesn't seem relevant to the patient's illness and isn't mentioned but is available in the comprehensive database.)

Personal/Social History, Lifestyle

Mrs. Jones works part time as a secretary as well as raising her three children. Her husband is employed by IBM. Mrs. Jones doesn't smoke, exercises daily, has a healthy diet, and generally leads a wholesome life. She has lived in this area all her life. There are no major family problems. She says the marriage is good. Her parents live nearby, and they can stay with the patient and look after the children. The family has adequate health insurance.

Discusses risk factors, which if present, might predispose to lung disease; general lifestyle, social support, and financial considerations which are relevant to care for the immediate problem.

☐ OBJECTIVE DATA

The patient, who is slender and quite pleasant, is uncomfortable but is ambulatory. She doesn't appear to be seriously ill. I judge her reliability to be excellent. She has a frequent dry cough. Her color is good; there is no cyanosis.

Your intuitive overall impression communicates a sense of how ill the patient is or how urgent the situation is. Sometimes a patient's general appearance tells more than any of the specific findings.

Vital Signs

Her temperature is 38° orally, pulse 95, blood pressure 115/75, and respirations 26 and a little shallow.

The fever suggests inflammation, the increased respiratory rate is consistent with a respiratory system disease. Height and weight are not relevant to this problem and are not mentioned.

Relevant Physical Findings

Ears, nose and throat are all negative.

Has a bearing on respiratory tract disease, but since there are no findings, only a brief "I've looked" statement is needed.

Examination of the chest shows definite splinting of the left side on deep breathing, no dullness but dry rales in the left base anteriorly and posteriorly. I've already mentioned her frequent dry cough. There is no abnormal fremitus.

Because the history suggested pulmonary disease it is important to give a complete report of this part of the examination.

The heart is negative except for the increased rate. There is no arrhythmia, abnormal heart sounds, or murmurs. There is no friction rub.

Because of the possibility of a heart disease causing the patient's symptoms, it is a good idea to report *in detail* pertinent negatives so the attending clinician knows exactly how thoroughly you examined the patient. To simply report a "negative heart exam" is less convincing and may raise questions such as "Did you specifically listen for a pericardial rub?"

Abdominal examination is normal.

Because chest pain occasionally arises from abdominal organs most clinicians would report at least briefly about this area.

The lower extremities were normal—no swelling, tenderness, change in temperature. The calf circumferences were equal.

> If you were concerned about a pulmonary embolus, this would be important "negative" information. If you hadn't considered this possibility, chances are the attending clinician would check the legs when examining the patient.

We obtained a complete blood count; the white blood count was 5600, and differential is normal. She was unable to raise sputum for a Gram's stain. The chest x-ray shows a patchy infiltrate in the left lower lobe. An EKG was normal.

□ ASSESSMENT

My assessment is that the patient has an inflammatory process in the left lower lobe of the lung. The normal white blood count and x-ray appearance are consistent with an infectious disease like mycoplasma or viral pneumonia, although a bacterial process cannot be excluded.

> Assessment is a brief statement of one's diagnostic thinking. Often the best one can do is identify the probable organ or system involved, the pathological process and weigh the relative significance of positive risk factors.

It is possible that she has some other primary problem in the left lower lobe such as tuberculosis, although this does not usually have an abrupt onset, and there are no risk factors. The patient is young for a neoplasm and is a non-smoker. A pulmonary embolus or a cardiac condition must be considered if more likely diagnoses are not confirmed.

□ PLANS

Regarding plans, further diagnostic testing should include sputum stain, acute phase cold agglutinin, and TB skin tests.

She has a supportive home situation and doesn't appear seriously ill; therefore, I believe she can be safely managed at home. Her husband or her parents can stay with her.

No specific treatment is indicated pending the lab studies or change in her condition. She should remain in bed, take fluids, and use a cough suppressant if the cough becomes fatiguing or interferes with sleep. While erythromycin might help shorten the illness, she tolerates oral antibiotics poorly and I don't think their use is essential.

> A straightforward statement of *all* therapy—not just medications.

Regarding patient education, I've explained the situation to her and her husband. I've mentioned possible complications and they know they can call us any time. If no problems arise, I'd like to see the patient in a week.

Identifies what the patient has been told. Documenting patient education is essential not only for the patient but also for other members of the health care team who may see the patient. This information is also valuable if a legal problem arises.

In Summary: The *Present Illness* suggested several possible systems (respiratory or cardiovascular). *Past Medical History, Family Medical History,* and *Personal* and *Social History* all contained some data that were *relevant;* data you judged not relevant are omitted. What is relevant depends to a great degree on seeing similar clinical problems in the past. Others who examine the patient might leave out or include other data, but you are presenting the clinical situation as you see it. The contributions of the attending physician and other members of the health care team guard against any errors you make; several examiners working together usually do a complete evaluation. The more experience you have, the better your sense of relevancy will be.

This brief example assumes you have a limited time to see the patient. Sometimes a patient's illness is too complex to be solved in the office. If she were sicker, hospitalization might have been warranted both for treatment and to permit obtaining a complete database.

☐ Additional Comments About Presentation Skills

When a patient has several active problems, start your presentation by mentioning all of the problems:

Mr. Brown is a 59-year-old man who has come to the clinic for two conditions—one, diabetes mellitus, and two, a slowly growing nodule on his face. First of all, regarding his diabetes. . .

After this initial statement, describe each problem separately in SOAP format.

☐ A Case Summary as Part of Rounds

When presenting a case summary as a part of formal rounds, where many professionals whom the patient doesn't know are present, several cautions apply. First, a patient's participation should be voluntary, not in any way forced. If the patient agrees to participate, explain the format of rounds: that health care professionals the patient doesn't know will be present, and that physical findings may be demonstrated.

Patients will wonder "Why me?" but may not come right out and ask. Some may think that something very serious has been discovered. Be sure patients know ahead of time just why they are being discussed. Without a clear explanation, their imagination may suggest all sorts of frightening reasons.

During the presentation, avoid jargon that the patient may misunderstand or misinterpret. If the patient is examined during the rounds, exposure must be as brief as possible.

After the presentation, return and ask if there are questions or concerns about what was discussed. Be sure your patient has not come away with misunderstandings about what was discussed.

Give some thought to the setting of the rounds. Will the appearance and behavior of those present reflect a professional environment? In some schools, eating lunch during rounds has become an accepted practice. Perhaps some patients don't mind or even notice, although it is difficult to see how eating while a patient's intimate concerns are discussed contributes to respectful setting.

A 30-year-old woman who suffered from headaches had been invited to noon-time rounds to be interviewed by a behavioral medicine specialist. Half of those present had brought lunch. Near the end of the interview, a fact emerged that had not previously been known: the patient's 5-year-old son had a slowly progressive, fatal blood disorder. The casual atmosphere of the rounds suddenly seemed quite inappropriate to the patient's situation.

It is common experience after you present a case that the attending physician learns from the patient important new information that you missed. Sometimes this results from the attending physician's greater experience of what to look for, but often your initial interview starts in motion a series of recollections which the attending physician "harvests." You do the work, the attending gets the credit!

Present the clinical material as you obtain it; don't bend the facts to fit a textbook picture.

Avoid stilted language: a "six-year-old female" is an impersonal way to describe a six-year-old girl. There is no need to dehumanize your description. Also, at times the patient is made to seem like someone in a court trial: you will frequently hear statements that the patient "denies" or the patient "admits" to having a certain symptom or having done some activity. What these words intend is giving listeners an idea of the accuracy of the information provided by the patient, but the impression may be created that the patient's truthfulness is questioned.

If a large number of laboratory tests are essential to your presentation (often they aren't), record them on a blackboard ahead of time, or prepare and distribute a summary sheet.

UNIT VIII

TECHNICAL SUPPORTS

CHAPTER 29

CHECKLISTS AND QUESTIONNAIRES

The interview, as a history-gathering tool, depends on memory in two respects:

1. The *interviewer* must remember to ask about several hundred items of information.

2. The *patient* is asked to recall health-related events which literally span a lifetime.

Medical care should not depend on memory. The human mind is not particularly good at precise recall of facts. Many variables influence the accuracy of memory at any one moment:

☐ Time since event.
☐ Fatigue.
☐ Stress and emotions.
☐ Information overload.

Checklists to help negotiate the intricacies of the medical interview are appropriate in a busy practice. Similarly, questionnaires to help patients recall health-related events of the past have a place in information-gathering. Both checklists and questionnaires, however, have limitations which must be understood if they are to be of maximal benefit in clinical practice.

☐ Checklists

Within the broad context of the *Fundamental Four* and the *Sacred Seven* are hundreds of items of specific information about your patients that you need to know. A Problem-Centered history is briefer than a Health Promotion interview, but even the briefest interview creates the opportunity for omission.

265

Sometimes, during a Problem-Centered interview you will find one area of the history so interesting that other areas are overlooked. In a Health Promotion interview, you face an information overload. The Review of Systems that accompanies *Chapter 7: The Review of Systems* lists more than 150 symptoms. However well prepared you are to interview a patient, you should not be expected to faultlessly remember the entire scope of a medical history.

A checklist cannot substitute for a thorough comprehension of the form and content of the history. It should not be a crutch, but a memory jogger that protects you against forgetting details of a task you know quite well. You cannot establish much of a relationship with a patient if you sit with your eyes on a checklist reading off questions. You need to focus most of your attention on the patient, and only occasionally glance at your checklist to ensure that you haven't overlooked something. A checklist can be a 3×5 card or a strip of paper affixed to a clip board.

Often the checklist will not make much of a difference in the accuracy of your history. It is under exceptional circumstances, when you are tired, or under time pressure, that omissions are most likely to occur. And it seems that significant mistakes happen just at the times when routines are abandoned and unexpected events occur.

The experience of the aviation regarding checklists has valuable lessons for the medical profession. Pilots, regardless of their years of experience, are required by law to use a checklist before every take-off and landing. Most of the time the procedure is automatic. But sooner or later a combination of circumstances makes a checklist critical.

A jet was taxiing to the runway. The take-off checklist had been completed when the plane was recalled to the terminal to pick up urgent cargo. One member of the crew retracted the flaps for the brief trip back to the terminal. As the plane returned to the runway for take-off the captain decided, contrary to company policy, that since he had just gone through the take-off preparations, he did not have to repeat the final check. The jet, lacking lift provided by the flaps, never got off the ground.

A checklist that guards against omission is just as appropriate when caring for patients as it is when flying an airplane.

☐ Patient-Administered Questionnaires

Compiling a database is time-consuming when done by direct interview. Regrettably, in today's increasingly expensive economic environment of medical practice, a detailed interview is the easiest procedure to omit to save time. One solution for gathering information is to use a questionnaire filled out by the patient. The patient can complete a questionnaire in a leisurely fashion at home, in contrast to the haste that may accompany the pressures of a busy practice. Often home records and family members provide information the patient has long since forgotten. Some patients may be more truthful in answering an impersonal questionnaire than they would be in a person-to-person interview, especially if guilt or shame is present. Questionnaires (paper or computer-based) may be the only practical way to obtain a medical history from deaf persons. Also, foreign language questionnaires are valuable in practices in which patients do not speak the language of the staff.

□ HEALTH DIARIES AND LISTS

Diaries perform a role similar to that of a questionnaire. They can be specific—a food diary for diet planning, for example—or they may be unstructured. Diaries are helpful in recording the circumstances of intermittent conditions such as episodes of heart rhythm irregularities. Self-reporting diaries may provide important insights into a patient's lifestyle, assuming the physician is willing to read what sometimes is lengthy prose (Verbrugge, 1980).

Some patients come to the doctor with lists of complaints. While sometimes an indication of hypochondriasis, such lists should be taken seriously and given careful scrutiny for both form and content (Burnum, 1985).

□ Questionnaire Limitations

While there are gains in using questionnaires, there are also losses. The patient's past life is more than a dry collection of facts. Feelings accompany past medical events. Sometimes the only way you can appreciate the full meaning of what the patient tells is by noting the way it is told.

Mr. Allen was a man in his 70's. He had long-standing diabetes mellitus with progressive peripheral vascular disease. He was hospitalized because of early gangrene of the left foot. The only procedure that would prevent the spread of the gangrene and the necessity for an amputation, was a vascular graft—not a particularly dangerous operation. When told of the need for the surgery, the patient refused to consider it. First the resident, then the attending physician, and finally the chief of surgery pleaded, argued, and finally threatened the patient, but without success. Finally, the staff decided the patient was mentally disturbed and asked for a psychiatric consultation.

The resident on psychiatry always repeated the Problem-Centered history before obtaining specialized psychological information. The patient's Past Medical History and Family Medical History were not remarkable. The first question of the Personal/Social history the resident asked was about the Mr. Allen's marital status. Mr. Allen said simply that his wife had died two years ago and that he was now living alone. Certainly not an exceptional fact for a man of his age. What was remarkable, and what would never have appeared on a questionnaire, was the way he answered. When he said simply, "My wife is dead," he paused, his voice lowered, and his eyes glistened with tears. His face reflected grief.

Further questioning about his wife brought out a story of coincidence, and the reason for refusing surgery. His wife had undergone surgery similar to that proposed for Mr. Allen, at the same hospital. She had died of complications. What the patient was thinking, but could not say to the surgeons, was "You killed my wife, but you are not going to kill me."

It would be nice to report that with the insight thus gained, the staff found a way to convince Mr. Allen that his wife's fate need not be his. But he did not have the surgery, and was transferred to a nursing home. His further history is not known.

No questionnaire can reflect the uniqueness of each patient, nor convey the nonverbal messages that are an essential part of the complete clinical experience. For this reason, some clinicians prefer to obtain all information by personal interview, despite the cost in personal time, because they believe that only in this way can they learn about the patient in depth. One such interview may go to the heart of a situation that frequent brief interviews will miss.

The variability of symptom terms is another limitation of questionnaires. The exact meaning of many of the words used to describe symptoms varies from patient to patient, as discussed in *Chapter 14: Verbal (Spoken) Communication*. Printed questionnaires cannot list the many alternative terms for the same symptom (although computer-based questionnaires have a "Do Not Understand" option; see the next chapter). Thus, an opportunity for misunderstanding exists, especially if the patient answers "No" to a symptom which is actually present.

A well-constructed questionnaire is not easy to prepare. In addition to the problems already mentioned, question sequence, the exact wording of a question, layout, and answer options influence questionnaire validity (Bennett and Ritchie, 1975).

Questionnaire use is not an "either an interview or a questionnaire" choice. Both have their strengths and limitations. My practice has been to have a new patient complete a comprehensive questionnaire before the initial visit. When I meet with the patient, I turn the questionnaire face down, and do a Problem-Centered interview. Only after completing the history do I look at the questionnaire. Occasionally, I learn new information that is relevant to the patient's problem. Mostly, however, the questionnaire provides factual information unrelated to the present problem but which is necessary to complete the comprehensive database.

□ Using Questionnaires During Medical School

As a student, using questionnaires or printed forms to obtain any part of the medical history would deprive you of the experiences needed to form your own style of data-gathering. As you proceed through a residency, you will have a chance to evaluate how you will use questionnaires. When entering practice is the time to make a decision on how much of your data-gathering effort you want to put into interviewing, and how much to leave to questionnaires or other history-taking methods.

□ REFERENCES AND READINGS

Bennett AE, Ritchie K: Questionnaires in Medicine: A Guide to Their Design and Use. London, Oxford University Press, 1975.

Burnum JF: La maladie du petite papier: Is writing a list of symptoms a sign of an emotional disorder? editorial. N Engl J Med 1985;313:691–692.

Verbrugge LM: Health diaries. Med Care 1980;XVIII:73–95.

CHAPTER 30

COMPUTERS AND INTERVIEWING

Modern medical practice is information intensive. Given the vast amount of health-related information, no clinician can be expected to rely on memory or sketchy records to practice quality, comprehensive care. The computer, as an information management instrument, can basically alter the way medicine is practiced.

☐ Rapport with a Computer?

The computer has achieved an impressive record in tasks based on "number crunching," but can a computer interview a patient? The computer is a machine: efficient, free of emotions or human warmth, dumb. Can such a device achieve the rapport or intelligence needed for a successful interview?

Experience with computer-based interviews suggests that people do relate to computers and will confide personal information. Slack (1984), a pioneer in computerized interviewing, describes the reactions of his first patient to participate in a computer interview:

> ... the patient seemed oblivious to his surroundings. He got going at the keyboard, responding to the questions appropriately, and after a while it became clear that there was a rapport between him and the machine. He laughed out loud at some of the comments from the computer. (Some I had intended to be funny; some I hadn't.) And he talked out loud to the machine, sometimes in praise and sometimes in criticism. "That was a dumb question," he noted with a chuckle. "You already asked me that!" He was right of course; it was my error ..., yet he never would have said this to me directly, a doctor with a white coat and a Bakelite name tag....

This man had *gained control*, not lost it. For the first time in his role as a patient he was in charge; he was master of this own history.

This interview focused on an emotionally neutral allergic history. Slack extended his studies to more sensitive areas, including gynecology and psychiatry, and found that patients are also willing to discuss intimate topics with computers. Indeed, some patients

> ... found themselves more comfortable in communicating information to the computer about potentially embarrassing matters, such as sexual activity, than they would have been talking to their physicians.

Another pioneer in the field of computer-human interaction, Weizenbaum, created ELIZA, a program that maintains a credible non-directive psychotherapeutic conversation. Weizenbaum (1976) reports:

> I was startled to see how quickly and how very deeply people became emotionally involved with the computer and how unequivocally they anthropomorphized it. Once my secretary, who had watched me work on the program for many months and therefore surely knew it to be merely a computer program, started conversing with it. After a few interchanges with it, she asked me to leave the room. Another time, I suggested I might rig the system so that I could examine all the conversations anyone had with it, say, overnight. I was promptly bombarded with accusations that what I proposed amounted to spying on people's most intimate thoughts. . . .

These observations suggest that interactive computers can play a role in effective psychotherapy. At the very least, the field is one that merits further research.

□ Computerized Interviewing

If people seem to develop a human-like relationship with some computers, does this mean the computer can go all the way—that it is just a matter of time and technical development before the entire interview will be safely entrusted to the computer? The answer, as you might guess, is somewhat in between an all-human and an all-computer interview. The challenge is determining the appropriate use of computers, and when their use is not suitable.

Computers are strongest in verbal communication skills. Yes/No questions, such as the *Review of Systems*, and limited-choice questions, are easy tasks for the simplest computers. More elaborate computer programs provide multiple "branches" to positive responses; elaborate branching programs simulate diagnostic reasoning.

In addition to prompting patients for factual information, computers can facilitate dialogue with responses like, "You are doing fine," or "I appreciate your telling me about that." Well-designed interviewing programs avoid the hazards of uncertainty about a question's meaning by offering the patient an "I don't understand the question" response, to which the computer can provide alternate terms or more detailed explanations. Patients interviewed by human practitioners do not always have the courage to say they don't understand a question or jargon. And at the conclusion of the interviews, the computer can summarize the history for the patient to review, and correct if necessary.

Free text entry is another matter. If the computer's response to a patient's statement is, "Tell me more about it," the patient may find it impossible to believe that the computer can understand sentences and paragraphs. Some computers do have a limited ability to make sense out of completely unstructured text, but this type of interpretive power is not really necessary. Most clinicians find a computer-generated report containing both the patient's free text and a summary of the patient's positive responses to the computer questionnaire a satisfactory, personalized document from which to work. Someday, perhaps, people will interact with computers in natural conversation: the computer asking questions with synthesized speech, and using speech recognition programs to record the patient's statements.

Nonverbal communication would seem to be out of bounds for a computer, but even here, interesting possibilities exist. While present-day computers cannot detect a tear or a frown, they can measure response times. In one program, if a delay (in terms of thousandths of a second) in keying in an answer is detected, the computer comments, "You seem to have difficulty answering that question. Do you want to discuss the subject in more detail?" Physiological responses such as a change in blood pressure, pulse, or galvanic skin resistance can be linked to the patient's response, although some persons might reasonably object that they are giving a medical history, not taking a lie detector test.

Computerized interviewing has other strengths. Computers are infinitely patient. Answers can be thoughtfully considered. The patient is under no subtle pressure to "hurry-up" as is often the case with a human interviewer who is behind schedule.

Interviewing programs are easily adapted to help persons with communication barriers such as deafness, blindness, or who understand only a foreign language. Persons with severe neuromuscular disabilities, such as quadriplegia, can interact with a computer through ingenious devices that detect direction of eye gaze, the slightest muscular contraction, a puff of air, or sucking. Even patients who are unable to read or recognize words because of brain damage (aphasia) can communicate through computer-generated pictures and symbols.

Costs of computer interviewing hardware and software are declining; in some situations they are competitive with the expense of an office visit to a practitioner.

Whatever the state of computer-based interviewing is when you begin to interview patients, you will be expected to compile the clinical database entirely by a conventional person-to-person interview. This is the only way you can develop the background necessary to make a sound judgment about the appropriate uses, as well as the limitations, of computers and other information tools you will employ in later years.

□ Decision Making

Throughout this book the diagnostic process has been presented as a skill capable of mastery by any thoughtful person. As more is learned about disease and its manifestations, the unaided mind will not be able to cope with the complexities of cognitive skills necessary for accurate diagnosis. The computer will be needed to assist in managing large amounts of data and complex diagnostic formulas.

Computer-based problem-solving employs three basic approaches:
1. Probabilistic/Statistical Methods.
2. Rule or Knowledge-based Programs.
3. Heuristics.

□ PROBABILISTIC/STATISTICAL METHODS

These diagnostic methods are based on a matching of a patient's illness with patterns of large numbers of past patients for whom the diagnosis is known. For example, the charts of hundreds of patients with abdominal pain who were found at surgery to have appendicitis are reviewed for the presence of symptoms, risk factors, physical findings, and laboratory tests. The data from this group of patients is gathered into a probability table indicating the likelihood of any clinical manifestation to be present in a patient with appendicitis. The clinical manifestations of the current, undiagnosed patient are matched against the known behaviors of past patients, and a probability score is constructed which expresses the chances that the patient has appendicitis. The process is like weather forecasting: when a forecaster says, "Today there is a 90 percent chance of rain," what is meant is that in past years at the same time, when conditions of temperature, barometric pressure, humidity, and other meteorology parameters were like those of today, it rained nine out of ten times.

For well-defined medical conditions like appendicitis, a predictive accuracy of 90 percent has been achieved. Notice that this approach does not depend on the *Disease = Location + Pathological Process + Cause* diagnostic approach used in this book. You only need to make accurate clinical observations and have accurate probability tables to achieve a high degree of diagnostic success. The interview, physical examination, and laboratory provide the data; after that the computer does the rest.

☐ RULE OR KNOWLEDGE-BASED PROGRAMS

Rule or knowledge-based decision support programs convert pragmatic knowledge of successful diagnosis and treatment into easily followed rules. No statistics are involved; rather, each problem is evaluated in terms of its characteristics. Often, all that is involved is making "yes/no" decisions about a series of specific decision-steps. In its simplest form, this approach resembles a game of twenty questions—each yes/no answer eliminates some possibilities, while other options are defined in ever greater detail.

A flow-chart or algorithm—the format this approach usually employs—specifies the kinds and sequence of clinical data that experience has shown to be the most effective in reaching the best decision. The sequence may be different than the traditional *Fundamental Four* approach. For example, a "lower abdominal pain" algorithm might specify as its very first question, "Have you been operated on for appendicitis?" An affirmative answer would eliminate one major line of subsequent investigation.

Another method of stating the decision-steps is by a series of "if . . . then" statements called production rules. These rules are arranged in order of increasing specificity: early questions are quite broad, later ones increasingly more focused.

Computers are essential for all but the simplest rule-based programs. Computers track many lines of investigation through dozens of decision points, a task the human mind cannot handle. Some rule-based programs have hundreds of rules and thousands of supporting literature abstracts. A book with this information would be so large and unwieldy that it would be impractical in a clinical setting.

☐ HEURISTICS

A third approach to clinical problems solving attempts to mimic the diagnostic thinking of expert physicians. *Heuristic* means "to discover" or "find one's way." Instead of starting with some preconceived idea of how the diagnostic process operates, this approach observes what experts actually do when problem-solving, whether the logic of their actions is evident or not. One such program, INTERNIST II, is able to successfully solve most of the clinicopathological case exercises of the *New England Journal of Medicine*. This project requires a mainframe computer; should the project reach a practical stage of operation, problem cases from all over the country could be brought to the computer by ordinary telephone communication techniques.

Major conceptual obstacles confront developers of expert programs.

Skilled, experienced diagnosticians often cannot explain exactly their mental processes while diagnosing a complex problem; the process is one that takes place on several psychological and cognitive levels simultaneously. No two patients may be approached in exactly the same way. The influence of nonverbal messages is not well appreciated. But active research continues and the limits of computer capabilities cannot be predicted.

The effort to develop expert programs has been successful in some diagnostic and therapeutic areas. These programs do not attempt to carry out the entire diagnostic process; rather they assist the physician in the various steps of the process by:

- ☐ Requesting and prompting for information a clinician may not think of obtaining.
- ☐ Retrieving relevant past information already in a database.
- ☐ Ensuring completeness of data gathering.
- ☐ Suggesting diagnostic possibilities based entirely on analysis of information, uninfluenced by the clinician's knowledge base, education, experience, or biases.
- ☐ Maintaining vigilance in repetitious, boring, or complex situations in which clinicians are subject to fatigue, diminished alertness, or information overload.

☐ Medical Records

The essential role of medical records in the health care process has been described in *Chapter 27: Medical Records.* In that chapter the record was viewed primarily as a passive means of recording clinical information. With the computer substituted for the traditional paper volume, the record becomes an active participant in the health care process, guiding the diagnostic and therapeutic processes. The references at the end of this chapter detail the capabilities of the computer record systems.

Only a few topics related to the interviewing process will be discussed here. For example, consider the importance of obtaining an accurate Past Medical History. When you stop to think about it, asking the patient for information about illnesses, hospitalizations, operations, and other events that occurred years or decades ago is expecting a great deal of the average person's memory. As time goes on, most people forget or distort such information. Furthermore, in many instances the patient may not have known the details of past medical episodes. In any event, the place to go to find such information is the original hospital record. If it is important to know the diagnosis and treatment about a heart condition that required hospitalization in 1975, the most accurate information would be obtained from the records of that hospitalization, rather than asking the patient for the details. The reason the patient is asked to supply the information is that old medical records are difficult to obtain. They may be stored on microfilm, or kept in a warehouse. Getting such records often takes weeks. Even if the patient's current chart contains information about events that occurred 10 or more years ago, the physician might have to search through hundreds or thousands of pages to locate needed information. I counted the pages of one such patient's chart: they numbered 3200 in eight separate volumes. Given these logistic obstacles, the only practical thing to do is ask the patient for the information, no matter how inaccurate it may be.

The only satisfactory solution to the problem of information storage and retrieval is to store it from the very beginning in a computer. Once in the computer, specific information, such as a report of an operation, can be obtained in a matter of seconds, or at most a few minutes. The technology for this type of information system has been available for years, although storing large amounts of rarely used information has been costly. The cost of mass storage has declined dramatically recently, and will continue to come down as new storage methods based on the laser are perfected.

Data input is a major bottleneck. Usually a physician dictates a note which is then passed to a clerk who enters the data into a chart or computer. This method is slow and costly, and introduces the chance of error. One solution is for physicians to learn enough typing skills that they can enter data directly into the computer. One commercially available system uses a small, light-weight (four pounds) portable computer that the physician carries into the examination room. The doctor enters a brief note while still with the patient, and the computer stores the information on a microcassette for later transfer to charts, or hospital records (Ash, 1983).

In Health Promotion, computers maintain constant surveillance over health maintenance programs. For example, a computer-based medical record system which has been in routine use for more than a decade on the Papago Indian Reservation near Tucson, Arizona, ensures that the following preventive medicine and general health measures are kept up-to-date:

☐ Blood tests for anemia.
☐ Immunizations.
☐ Vision and hearing evaluations.
☐ Growth and development of children.
☐ Tuberculosis screening.
☐ Pap testing for women.
☐ Family planning services.

These parameters are displayed every time a patient comes for care for any condition, so that Problem-Centered and Health Promotion services can be provided at the same time. Furthermore, the patient's records are available wherever the patient appears for care (there are three clinics and a hospital scattered over an area the size of Rhode Island).

Other clinical benefits of computer-based records include:

□ Making information available to all health care personal when and where needed, without waiting in line for someone else to finish using the traditional record.
□ Enabling accurate audit of information as a part of a quality-of-care program.
□ Alerting of potential risks, such as ordering penicillin for someone with a past history of a penicillin reaction.
□ Detecting pattern of illness, such as a beginning epidemic, in a community.
□ Providing legible copies of the record to the patient, along with computer-generated patient information materials.
□ Assisting in cost control efforts.

Despite the many benefits of computer-based records, they are not likely to be widely used until there is an awareness by the medical profession of the inadequacy of the traditional medical record, and the enormous direct and indirect costs of trying to provide modern health care with an information system that is essentially the same as it was 50 years ago.

□ Patient Education

Computers are easily adaptable to a variety of patient education services. Online database services like *CompuServe* have programs that provide users with access to health care professionals (Conroy, 1986). An electronic bulletin board, originally intended for physicians, has been adopted by patients seeking advice on a wide range of topics (Grundner and Garrett, 1986). And the CD-ROM, with its ability to store and rapidly access hundreds of thousands of text on a single 4.72 inch disk, makes available enormous libraries of health-related information.

□ Confidentiality

Protecting the confidentiality of information in computer systems is an understandable concern, and one reason why physicians are cautious about changing over to the computerized records. But current methods of handling records provide little protection against unauthorized use. Charts are often left unattended in a hospital or clinic for any curious person to look at. In some hospitals, anyone with a white coat or stethoscope could, by simple deception, obtain a records. In Illinois a few years ago, attorneys looking for malpractice cases obtained records by bribing low-paid record clerks. Computers, while not totally free of security abuses, are protected by electronic locks, passwords,

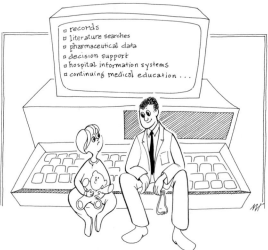

The computer can liberate the physician
to exercise uniquely human skills.

and other safety measures. They provide a far safer system for protecting confidential information than do present methods.

☐ Clinical Research

Research implies universities, technicians, and huge computers. But clinical research can also be done by any practitioner who keeps orderly patient records. Opportunities for research exist within any kind of practice. In one dramatic instance, a practitioner noted in his practice the presence of a rare form of liver cancer at a rate far above what would be expected in the population he served. This observation lead to detection of a major health hazard in a nearby chemical plant. Other clinical research studies carried out in clinical settings included:

☐ Age/sex distribution of illnesses.
☐ Utilization of health care resources.
☐ Patterns of prescribing psychotropic drugs.
☐ Effectiveness of preventive medicine measures.
☐ Natural history of common disease.
☐ Evaluation of therapies for obesity.
☐ New drug evaluation studies.

Until recently, such studies were carried out with nothing more than well-organized records. With the availability of powerful microcomputers and flexible software, large amounts of primary data can be analyzed with the same speed previously available only in mainframe computers. The rapidly expanding area of outpatient medicine, particularly, has had very little study compared to hospital-based research.

□ Computers and Humanism

Critics of computer-assisted medical practice suggest the human touch will be lost, that medical care will be impersonal and sterile. I believe the opposite is the case. At present, physicians are trying to manage enormous amounts of clinical information in their heads, aided by an archaic information and record system. As medicine becomes more complex, the amount of technical information the clinician is responsible for increases. There is only so much time for a clinician to spend with each patient, and the technical usually demands priority over the interpersonal aspects of care detailed in this book. Until the profession recognizes the impossibility of keeping up with its vast information load, and is willing to turn much of the technical side of medical practice over to the computer, physicians will not have the time needed to interact with patients as one human to another.

No computer will ever detect the subtleties of interaction between clinician and patient that occur in the examining room or at the bedside. The computer can liberate the physician to exercise these uniquely human skills while, at the same time, placing complex diagnostic and therapeutic decisions on a far more accurate, dependable, and scientific basis than is now the case.

□ REFERENCES AND READINGS

Blum, BI (ed): Information Systems for Patient Care. New York, Springer-Verlag, 1984.

Bursztajn H, Feinbloom R, Hamm RM, et al: Medical Choices, Medical Chances, New York, Dell/Seymour Lawrence, 1981.

Conroy C: Online lifeline. Online Today 1986;5:14–18.

Erdman HP, Griest JH: Direct patient computer interviewing. J Consult Clin Psychol 1985;53:760–773.

Grundner TM, Garrett RE: Interactive medical telecomputing. An alternative approach to community health education. New Engl J Med 1986;314:982–985.

Levinson D: Information management in clinical practice. J Fam Pract 1978;7:799–805.

Levinson D: Information, computers, and clinical practice. JAMA 1983;249:607–609.

Levinson D: Computer Applications in Clinical Practice: An Overview. New York, Macmillan, 1985.

Redman RW, Everett GD, Wallace RB: Research in family medicine. In Rakel RE (ed): Textbook of Family Practice, ed 3. Philadelphia, WB Saunders Co, 1984, Chap 24.

Slack WV: A history of computerized medical interviews. M.D. Computing 1984; 1:52–59.

Weizenbaum J: Computer Power and Human Reason: From Judgment to Calculation. San Francisco, WH Freeman and Company, 1976, pp 6–7.

Ziporyn T: Medical decision making: Analyzing options in the face of uncertainty. JAMA 1983;249:2133–2142.

A PROBLEM-CENTERED INTERVIEW

The patient, a 47-year-old man, was making the first visit to the office where he was interviewed. Even though he had no appointment, a careful assessment of his current problem—chest discomfort—was essential, since chest pain is always of concern and sometimes an emergency. Situations like this, where time to see a patient must be created in an already busy schedule, are typical of the challenges in a busy medical practice.

This type of interview, although brief, is in many ways more demanding than is a lengthy one to obtain a comprehensive history. Every question must serve a diagnostic or therapeutic purpose. There is no place for "routine" questions. Also, because of the time constraints and the possibility that the patient's initial complaint might indicate a serious illness, Health Promotion questions are omitted.

This interview incorporates the principles detailed in *Unit II: Problem-Solving* and some of the techniques described in *Unit IV: Communication Techniques*. As you read through it, try to decide what *organs/systems* are likely to be involved; *Think Organs/Systems* rather than trying to identify what disease is present. Note the various interviewing techniques used. Finally, you should appreciate that the transcript conveys very little of the nonverbal information that in an actual interview adds substantial information.

☐ Transcript

Mr. Loomis is white and about 30 percent overweight. He walked into the clinic looking tense and pale, but not seriously ill. He was sweating, but the day was hot and humid.

Mr. Loomis?

Yes.

I am Dr. Swanson. I am a family doctor with the clinic. How can I help you today? (Interviewer's name and role identified.)

Well, for the past week-and-a-half I have been having a burning sensation in my chest, and it has been getting worse as time goes on.

I see. . . a pain in your chest?. . . a burning sensation. . . ? (Repeating the patient's last words to encourage him to continue the broad overview.)

Yes. I have been taking Tums for it. I think it is something to do with my stomach, and Tums have seemed to relieve it for awhile. For the last two days the sensation gets worse as I walk.

I see. Is there anything else you can tell me about it? (Open-ended technique to encourage the patient to continue his unstructured narrative.)

The sensation was getting more and more severe. I was pretty sure that I could take care of it by myself. I am pretty sure it is not a heart condition or anything like that (laughs). I just thought it was a bug. I am new to town. I am an architect. Today I have had to do a lot of walking back and forth and my wife has been after me to see a doctor. So I said as soon as I can I will go to the clinic.

So it is getting gradually worse?

Well, it was a little more acute than that. Today it was quite bad. I took a bus in today and it is about a half-mile, but I couldn't make it all the way without stopping. And this has never happened before. . . I had to sit down on the way in.

How are you feeling right now? (An interruption to decide if the patient's condition warrants urgent intervention or whether it is safe to continue and obtain more information, which would make patient care more specific.)

Right now I can feel it but I am comfortable.

Let me ask you a few more questions. You describe this as a "burning sensation" in the center of your chest? Can you show me exactly where it is? (Beginning of the *Sacred Seven* analyzing the symptom of chest pain.)

Right about here (points to the sternal area).

And does it go any place else?

It is hard for me to localize pain, but I'm pretty sure this one stays pretty much here.

Any sensation anywhere else (pause)—arms, neck, shoulders, jaws?

No.

And the *quality* of this sensation is a "burning?"

That is as well as I can describe it.

How *severe*, how bad is it?

Well, suppose if you pushed here (presses on his sternum) as hard as you could, I think it would be like that.

How about stubbing your toe—is it that bad?

Oh, no (laughs) that is much worse.

Well, if you took "ten" as the worse possible pain and freedom from pain as "zero," could you give this a rating?

Oh, at its worst, I would say between "five" and "six."

You mentioned that this has been present for a week-and-a-half. . . (Chronology/Timing.)

It might have been present longer than that, but I just discounted it because it was so mild. . .

How often did it come at first?

I can't say, but it has been really noticeable in the last three or four days.

In any event, there has been a progression in the frequency. . .

Yes.

And what were you doing when this first started? (Onset/Setting.)

Nothing special.

Any event you could relate to the onset?

No.

You said you had just come to town.

Yes, we came from the East, and we pulled a trailer.

How long ago was that?

A week-and-a-half ago.

So, just upon your coming to town you started having difficulties.

(Pause) . . . Yes (thoughtfully), . . . that is right.

In terms of making this better for you, you mentioned Tums. . . is there anything else that relieves it?

Not that I can think of.

You also mentioned that if you stop what you are doing, that relieves the pain?

Yes, that is the best!

Is there anything else that aggravates it?

No.

Eating, does that make any difference?

I'm not sure. I'd like to say that it does, but I'm not sure.

Let me summarize the problem as I understand it right now. A week-and-a-half ago you came to town and about that time you experienced what you describe as a burning sensation about the center of your chest. . . (Summarization provides the interviewer a chance to confirm his understanding thus far, and gives the patient a chance to add or correct information. Also this is a good time for the interviewer to make notes before continuing.)
. . . and that you describe it as five on a scale of ten. And it is severe enough when you get it that you have to stop what you are doing. It is becoming gradually more frequent until yesterday and today you have been having it almost steadily.

It is only in the past two or three days that I have had to stop, really stop, what I have been doing.

And the setting of this is that this started just as you arrived in town, but you don't remember exactly what you were doing when the onset of the first episode. . .

That's right.

And that things like Tums may make a bit of difference, but what really helps now is stopping what you are doing.

In the past few days I am sure Tums are not making any difference although before they were.

Are there any other symptoms you are having along with this pain?

Well, I do have some wheezing, I don's think it is related in any way. I do have a history of allergy and I take Chlortrimeton (an antihistamine medication) at times to relieve the wheezing. . .

Have you tried any Chlortrimeton to relieve this condition?

Yes.

And did it make any difference?

No.

Are there any other symptoms that might come from your lungs? Cough? . . . sputum . . . wheezing . . . chest pains when you take a deep breath . . . shortness of breath . . .?

Yes.

Tell me about that.

Well, even when the burning sensation was mild, if I took a very deep breath, I could feel it, but is was very slight.

You mentioned the heart. Are there any other symptoms that might indicate something abnormal with your heart?

No, as a matter of fact I am convinced that it is not my heart. I have been told that my heart is as strong as an ox (laughs).

Any palpitations . . . irregular heart beat . . . any sweating or feeling of weakness . . . ankle swelling . . . circulation trouble . . .? (Even though the patient cannot think of any cardiovascular symptoms when first asked, the interviewer is sufficiently concerned about this system that he decides to evaluate it in detail. Had the doctor felt this system was unlikely to be involved, he might have been satisfied to ask the single open-ended question, "How about your heart and circulation?" Similar considerations apply to the gastrointestinal system which is investigated next.)

No.

How about your stomach and digestion?

Very good.

Any bad taste in the mouth . . . difficulty swallowing . . .nausea . . . belching . . . cramps or abdominal pains . . . change in bowel habits— diarrhea or constipation . . . gas . . . significant weight change?

No.

. . . Is there anything else about this present problem that I haven't asked about?

Not that I can think of.

Now before I examine you, let me get an idea about your past medical history. (Transitional question.) How has your health been in the past?

Very, very good. The only time I was in the hospital was in the service, and that was a minor thing—they called it nasopharyngitis.

Any serious illnesses or under the care of a doctor for a long period of time?

No.

In the hospital for anything other than the nasopharyngitis—any operations or injuries?

No.

Are you taking any medicines regularly?

Yes. I have quite a few headaches, and there are times I take a lot of aspirin.

What do you mean by a lot of aspirin? (Documentation.)

Oh, perhaps nine tablets a day.

Have you been taking aspirin at that rate recently?

No . . . not as much aspirin as I have taken in the past.

Ever have trouble taking aspirin—stomach distress or abdominal pain? (This inquiry is based on aspirin's ability to cause gastric irritation, which can be felt as chest discomfort similar to the patient's "heartburn.")

No.

Are you taking other medications?

No.

Any allergies to medicines? (Anticipation of a treatment plan and the need to avoid any drugs to which the patient is sensitive.)

No.

Now, I'd like to ask about your family's health. (Transitional question.) How is the health in your family?

I have one brother who is in good health. I have a son, he is very healthy. My parents are both dead. They died in the past four years.

What did your mother die of?

Technically it was called heart failure. She did have angina, I think they called it.

And your father?

My father died technically of heart failure, but at the time he was undergoing a progressive nerve disease.

And did he have an angina?

It is hard to say (pause), but I get the impression that he did have angina. (Patient lightly touches the cheek just below his right eye. This nonverbal gesture, which appears like brushing away a tear, is commonly indicative of sadness. Watch for this fleeting gesture.)

Are there any other illnesses that run in the family?

No.

Now, I'd like to know more about you. You explained that you are an architect and have recently come to town. You are married and have a son. Can you tell me about yourself?

What would you like to know?

Do you smoke?

No, I never have.

How would you describe your diet?

I think it is very well balanced. My wife makes me eat well.

How about fatty foods, and rich foods like ice cream?

We hardly ever have fried foods. I do like ice cream but don't overdo it.

What do you do for recreation?

Lately, I haven't done anything except move.

Do you exercise regularly?

No, and I have a big waistline to prove it.

What about health insurance—sometimes when you make a change in a working situation, insurance can be a real problem?

I thought about that before moving. Fortunately, I was able to continue the Blue Cross.

Is there anything else you can think of at this point?

No . . . Yes, there is one more thing. About ten years ago I was having some pain in my stomach. They took some x-rays, but they weren't conclusive. They thought I might have an ulcer, and they suggested I have some other tests. And I asked them what would happen if I took the other tests and I did have an ulcer? They said they would put me on a special diet. So I said, why don't you put me on the special diet and see what happens? And they did, and I found I felt even worse, so I gradually discontinued the diet and the pain gradually went away.

Was the pain anything like what you are experiencing now?

No.

You have already told me that you do not think this is heart trouble—what do you think it could be?

Well, I thought it was a "bug" that is going around.

Is there anything you would like to ask me right now?

No, I cannot think of anything.

Well, let's go in the examining room. I'll have some other questions to ask during the examination, and maybe you'll think of other things, too . . .

The examination was essentially normal. However, an electrocardiogram taken in the office showed abnormalities consistent with cardiac ischemia. The patient was therefore transferred to a hospital cardiac monitoring unit, where over several days he became symptom-free and his electrocardiogram returned to normal. One week following hospital admission, at 2 a.m., the patient experienced a major myocardial infarction and cardiac arrest. By a fortunate coincidence, a cardiologist was in the room examining another patient and was able to resuscitate Mr. Loomis.

The patient lost weight and lived a productive life, which included creative employment and world-wide travel. He developed mild diabetes mellitus about ten years following the myocardial infarction. Thirteen years following his infarction, at age 65, he died in his sleep.

□ Comments

Note the amount of information contained in the initial, unstructured question: the initial symptom, the recent move, the patient's occupation, that he is married, and his impression of what is causing the illness.

Early in the interview, the interviewer has raised several *organ/system* possibilities: a *cardiac* condition (based on symptom analysis), upper *gastrointestinal* disease (early relief from Tums, and the risk factors of high aspirin intake and questionable past history of ulcer). *Respiratory* disease would be a distant third, since neither the main symptom (the "very slight" chest pain on deep breathing) nor the wheezing history seems significant. This, however, is more of an intuitive than a rational judgment. The relevant *Review of Systems* was then used during the *Associated Symptoms* questioning (the seventh component of the *Sacred Seven*) to further narrow the range of possible *organs/systems*.

Notice the constant alternation between open-ended and forced choice questions in every stage of the interview. For example, "How has your health in the past been?" . . . "Have you ever been in the hospital?"

At the conclusion of the interview, no organ/system diagnosis has been made with certainty. As new lines of information emerged during the interview, the weight of evidence shifted between the possibilities. What had been achieved was a narrowing of organ/system possibilities. The physical examination and laboratory testing remain to be done, and may (or may not) achieve a disease diagnosis.

The sequence of the interview is not strictly logical. The question of the ulcer was brought up long after the interviewer had left the *Past Medical History.*

Throughout the interview the patient answered in precise terms, often attempting to reach an impractical degree of precision. What type of personality pattern fits this patient? Are there certain occupations that attract such persons? Are there implications for treatment implied in the personality assessment of your patients?

The relevant system reviews can take up a lot of time if each symptom is asked as a question: "Have you any cough?" "Do you bring up sputum?" "Have you any wheezing?" The economical way to get through a system review is simply to name the symptom, followed by a brief pause: "Any cough . . . sputum . . . wheezing . . . ?"

Denial of the possibility of serious disease is evident at several points in the interview. Can you identify the patient's statements and behaviors that support this impression?

The interchange about the *onset/setting* of the patient's illness represents an *interpretation*—namely, the illness began in the setting of a major life change. While relevant to the interviewer's professional interests, the topic was not relevant to the patient's immediate needs, and was not discussed further at this point. Had the patient been acutely ill, the question would not have been raised at that time.

This transcript is based on a taped interview of the patient, but has been edited and altered to highlight interviewing principles. For a complete, unedited interview, see Morgan and Engel: *A Clinical Approach to the Patient.* Philadelphia, W.B. Saunders Co., 1969, pp 243–281.

INDEX

Note: Numbers in *italics* refer to illustrations; numbers followed by (t) refer to tables; numbers followed by (n) refer to footnotes.